Problems in
Social Care

Problems in Practice Series

Problems in Practice Series

Series Editors : J.Fry K.G.D.Williams M.Lancaster-Smith

Problems
in
Social Care

Roslyn H. Corney
PhD, Dip. App. Soc. Studies

Lecturer
General Practice Research Unit
Institute of Psychiatry
London

1983 **MTP PRESS LIMITED**
a member of the KLUWER ACADEMIC PUBLISHERS GROUP
BOSTON / THE HAGUE / DORDRECHT / LANCASTER

Published by
MTP Press Limited
Falcon House
Lancaster, England

Copyright © 1983 R.H. Corney
Softcover reprint if the hardcover 1st edition 1983
First published 1983

British Library Cataloguing in Publication Data

Corney, Roslyn H.
 Problems in social care–(Problems in practice
 series)
 1. Social problems
 I. Title II. Series

 361.1   HN18

ISBN-13: 978-94-009-6588-1   e-ISBN-13: 978-94-009-6586-7
DOI: 10.1007/978-94-009-6586-7

Contents

Contents

Preface

This book has been written primarily for general practitioners; it describes the social problems which are presented by patients to their doctors for help and advice. The aim of the book is to help the doctor manage these problems, both through his own interventions and by involving or referring the patient on to other agencies.

While the more common problems have been considered in detail, those rarely encountered have been omitted. The book also concentrates on help available from non-medical sources, as these will be less familiar to the general practitioner than other medical or nursing services.

There is often a close association between social difficulties and health problems, both physical and psychiatric. It is, therefore, vital that an attempt is made to meet the social needs of patients in order to promote good physical and mental health.

R.H. Corney

Series Foreword

This series of books is designed to help general practitioners. So are other books. What is unusual in this instance is their collective authorship; they are written by specialists working at district general hospitals. The writers derive their own experience from a range of cases less highly selected than those on which textbooks are traditionally based. They are also in a good position to pick out topics which they see creating difficulties for the practitioners of their district, whose personal capacities are familiar to them; and to concentrate on contexts where mistakes are most likely to occur. They are all well-accustomed to working in consultation.

All the authors write from hospital experience and from the viewpoint of their specialty. There are, therefore, matters important to family practice which should be sought not within this series, but elsewhere. Within the series much practical and useful advice is to be found with which the general practitioner can compare his existing performance and build in new ideas and improved techniques.

These books are attractively produced and I recommend them.

J.P. Horder CBE
Past President, The Royal College
of General Practitioners

1 Social problems: the key role of the doctor

Close association between health and social problems

It has long been recognized that the individual in society must be seen in the context of his social enviroment. Thus, the social and psychological components of physical and mental illness are vital and may be in some cases as important as the biological components. Poverty and poor housing, for example, have a demonstrably detrimental effect on physical and mental health while problems in personal relationships or a life crisis such as a bereavement frequently cause psychological distress. In addition to social problems affecting physical or mental health, illnesses or disabilities can directly affect a person's social circumstances. Someone who becomes physically disabled may lose his job, his wife may leave him, thus making him poor and lonely. Indeed, the problems of living with the chronic diseases are medicosocial and appropriate medical help has to take into account the physical, mental and social effects of these illnesses.

Major part of the doctor's workload

As patterns of health need have changed, the workload and role of the general practitioner has radically altered. Nervous system disorders, social and emotional problems are now the second most common category of reason for attending a general practitioner after coughs, colds and upper respiratory tract infections. One survey conducted in Buckinghamshire ably demonstrated the psychosocial content of the general practitioner's work. Seventy doctors were asked to give standardized information about every patient seen on a certain day. Replies indicated that over one third of patients were believed by the doctor to have or cause some social or psychosocial difficulty. Four main social problem areas were identified with four

11

groups of patients, the mentally ill and handicapped, the elderly, the physically disabled or chronically ill and those patients with marital and sexual problems.

The changing pattern of illness

There are a number of reasons why the psychosocial component of the doctor's workload has increased in recent years. First, the numbers of elderly and handicapped in the community has risen dramatically, thus increasing those who need a disproportionate amount of medical and social help. This is due in part to the dramatic decline in infectious

More handicapped and elderly patients in the community

diseases which previously caused many people to die at a young age. Other successes of medicine have kept alive malformed babies and accident victims which also increases the numbers of handicapped. There has also been a shift against caring for the elderly and handicapped in hospitals towards keeping them at home or in local authority establishments. This transfers the responsibility of caring for these groups from hospitals to community health and social services.

Secondly, there has been a growing trend for people to look for medical answers to their social and emotional problems.

Increasing 'medicalization' of social problems

Patients may present a whole range of problems which would not have previously been regarded as medical matters. They may present an overt social problem with no medical content or, alternatively, a health problem or minor symptom, hoping that the underlying social difficulty will be brought up and discussed.

It has been found that people with social problems are more likely to contact their doctor than any other social service and there are a number of reasons for this. Most people are registered with a general practitioner, have visited him on several occasions and find his surgery accessible. Other social agencies may be inaccessible or unfamiliar to the patient or he may not even know of their existence. Increased geographical mobility means that many people do not live close to family

Reasons why people visit their doctor

or friends and so may have no one to confide in other than their family doctor.

In addition, health problems have greater social acceptability than emotional or personal ones and patients find that attending a doctor with an 'illness' or a 'symptom' is more

More socially acceptable

acceptable to both themselves and others than visiting someone specifically for a social problem. The general practitioner may also prescribe drugs to relieve psychological distress which may be another influential factor in determining whose help will be sought.

It follows, therefore, that an appreciable amount of a general practitioner's time will be spent in dealing with social problems, often occurring in conjunction with ill health.

Doctor's role is of vital importance

How the doctor spends this time is of vital importance, as it has been widely recognized that the social relationship between patient and doctor can have a powerful therapeutic effect. It has been estimated, for example, that as much as a third of the success of any drug or procedure may be attributable to this relationship (the placebo effect). Thus, how the doctor handles the patient's social and psychological problems may play a major role in determining whether the problem is eventually resolved.

The doctor's ability to help, however, is handicapped by the poor link between health and social welfare services. Recently, the Social Services Act created a community service from the old Welfare, Children's and Mental Health departments.

Split between health and welfare services

However, this has, in general, brought about an even greater separation between medical and social services.

One of the aims of this book is to suggest ways in which the doctor can try to help the social and psychological problems presented to him by his patients, both by his own interactions and by enlisting the involvement and support of other agencies. It is hoped that it will provide a guide to the extensive statutory and voluntary services available to those in need.

The social services and sources of help for social problems

This chapter will give a brief outline of the main local services available to help those with social problems and difficulties. The addresses and phone numbers of these local agencies will be available by contacting the town hall or through the telephone directory.

Local authority social services department

Services, day-care and residential provision

These departments carry out a number of services, many of which are statutory. They provide help for all sections of the community, children, young adults, the middle-aged and the old. As well as supplying services in the home, local authorities provide day-care facilities and residential accommodation for a number of groups in need, including children, the elderly, the physically and mentally ill and disabled.

Types of help given

The field work staff of social services departments, called social workers, are usually based in teams covering a specific area. These social workers deal with a wide range of social problems, although some local authorities employ specialist social workers for the blind and the deaf. Social workers play a key role in arranging adoptions, fostering, registering and supervising child-minders, juvenile court work and child care proceedings, including those where children have been neglected or abused. They also provide help for the elderly and handicapped, including services such as meals-on-wheels, home helps, day-care and employment facilities for the dis-

15

abled, and residential accommodation. Social workers will
also give advice or undertake counselling as well as providing
practical help and services. In general, if a social worker is
unable to help with a particular problem, she will suggest an
alternative agency who can.

*Counselling
undertaken*

The address of the local area team can be obtained from the
town hall. In many cases, however, the patients of a practice
will be covered by more than one area team depending on their
geographical boundaries. Some local authorities, however, are
favourable towards the idea of attaching social workers to general practice so that one particular social worker receives all the
referrals from the practice. Thus, some local authorities may
welcome an approach by a general practitioner to this effect.

*Address from
the town hall*

*Social work
attachment*

Social workers are also employed by medical and psychiatric
departments in hospitals. Although they generally assist
with a patient's problems while he is in hospital, they will
sometimes stay involved after discharge, especially in the case
of mental illness.

*Medical and
psychiatric
social workers*

Local authority housing departments

Some local authorities have set up housing advisory services,
for people in all types of accommodation who have a housing
problem or query. In addition, the local authority housing
department provides council housing and has the responsibility to house certain groups, such as the disabled or families
who are genuinely homeless. Other local authority departments employ rent and rent tribunal officers who will decide
on a 'fair rent' for privately rented accommodation. Details of
all these services can be obtained from the town hall.

*Housing
services*

Local education authority

This is the body responsible for providing educational facilities. The Special Education Service is concerned with providing facilities for children with various handicaps, including the
maladjusted and the physically or mentally handicapped.

*Special
Education
Service*

The welfare of all school age children is the responsibility of
the Education Welfare Service. Education welfare officers
(EWOs) carry out a wide range of duties ranging from many
administrative tasks to counselling. They can be involved in
cases where the school child exhibits behaviour problems or

The EWO

16

fails to attend school, where there are difficulties in communication between teachers and parents or where the family has financial or transport problems hindering school attendance. Normally, EWOs have large caseloads so are unable to offer intensive work with any one family.

The area health authority – the health visitor

Although the duties of health visitors include responsibilities towards the mentally and physically handicapped and elderly, most health visitors consider their main role is to assist the families of children under 5 years. However, because their roles and functions are so diverse, there is a considerable variance among health visitors according to whether they regard dealing with social problems as a major part of their role. Generally, those health visitors who work closely with general practitioners in an attachment scheme of some kind have extended the social component of their work. In these situations, they may act in a similar manner to a social worker, giving advice, guidance and involving other relevant agencies.

Child guidance

These clinics vary considerably in the type of work carried out. Many still give individual help and treatment to families
Treatment and advice with preschool or school age children, while others act more as consultants to the education departments, juvenile courts, community homes, etc.

The probation and aftercare service

There has been a shift over the last few years for the local authority social services department to take on a greater responsibility for juvenile court work and for the probation
After care support for adult offenders officers to develop their work with adults, especially aftercare support for those released from detention centres, borstals and prisons. They also engage in helping the families of prisoners.

Matrimonial work Another important role of the probation officer is matrimonial work. Individuals with marital difficulties can approach their local probation officer for counselling and help. Probation officers are often involved in court cases where there

17

are matrimonial disputes and are called upon to act as independent assessors.

Department of Health and Social Security (local offices)

There is a local office for every area and these offices are responsible for handling the state benefits such as pensions, sickness benefits and supplementary benefits. Staff of these offices can also help in an emergency or in cases of real financial hardship. Claimants can apply at their local office and will be given details of the various benefits to which they may be eligible. In addition, post offices also have leaflets describing certain benefits, sometimes with an application form attached.

The state benefits

Help in an emergency

Department of Employment (local employment offices or job centres)

The staff of employment offices give details of job vacancies, advice on employment and careers, and provide specialist services for the disabled and others. They can also give information on government training courses and schemes, including the Youth Opportunities Programme (YOP). The unemployed can claim their benefit from unemployment offices.

Information, advice and law centres

Local authority information centres

Some local authorities provide information centres which are often situated in the town hall or other council offices. Some authorities also employ welfare rights officers who are familiar with the complexities of the welfare and social security system and can give advice and guidance.

Information centres

Citizens' advice bureaux

There are more than 700 of these bureaux in Britain which means that most towns and all the big cities have at least one. These bureaux offer a general information and advisory service which anyone can use for any query. In certain

General advisory service

cases, the staff will also act on an individual's behalf. If unable to help, the staff will give the names and addresses of more suitable agencies, such as lawyers, counsellors or social workers.

Up-to-date knowledge

Although the majority of the staff are voluntary, they are given training and are provided with up-to-date information about legislation, social service and relevant material, including local issues. Many offices have specialist sessions engaging experts in legal, financial, welfare rights, housing and consumer affairs.

Legal advice and law centres

There are a number of centres (especially in the large cities) which give legal advice. Although there are fewer law centres, the lawyers in these not only give advice but will handle cases from start to finish. These agencies are run either by the local authority or by voluntary organizations, and normally services are free.

The role of voluntary organizations

The role of voluntary agencies

Voluntary agencies play a major part in providing help and services to those with social difficulties. Although the services provided by the state have increased dramatically during this century, there is still such a large gap between social need and statutory provision that there is a great need for voluntary effort.

Increase the choice available

The services provided by voluntary bodies often supplement those provided by the statutory agencies, covering the same range but increasing the choice available. For example, voluntary organizations provide residential accommodation for the elderly and handicapped, special schooling, hostels and day centres. Often in these cases, the voluntary bodies set up the facilities but the majority of the costs are met by the local authority.

Provide additional services

In addition, voluntary bodies often provide a range of services beyond the scope of the statutory agencies. They can provide volunteers to visit the elderly and do jobs such as gardening or decorating. Other voluntary agencies give intensive counselling help to deprived families. In some circumstances, voluntary bodies are the sole providers of services, especially when new needs arise.

19

The relative independence of voluntary agencies conveys a number of advantages. They have much more freedom than the statutory bodies and can thus use innovatory and pioneering methods. They can also criticize the statutory agencies and question government policy. In recent years, there has been an increase in the number of agencies run on the 'self-help' principle. These groups are wholly or largely run by their own members. Thus, people with problems in common can resolve their difficulties by helping each other and providing mutual support.

Unfortunately, voluntary provision is very uneven across different geographical areas and with different types of need. However, details of the voluntary bodies operating in each area can be obtained from the local council of social service or voluntary service. These councils try to co-ordinate the voluntary efforts in their area and should have lists of local groups. Details of voluntary agencies can also be obtained from the National Council of Social Services (for address, see Appendix 1).

Have more
independence

Self-help
groups

Council of
social service

③ Children and young people

This chapter covers some of the problems faced by children as well as some of the services and help developed to overcome them. Certain family problems are covered in other chapters, for example, the financial problems of families are included in the chapter on finance while adoption and fostering are included in the chapter on adult and family life.

Behaviour problems in children

Most children exhibit some behaviour disturbances at certain times. They may have problems sleeping or eating, they may have temper tantrums or breathholding attacks. They are likely to regress into babyish behaviour at certain times, especially at the arrival of a new baby.

Common occurrence

In most cases where the behaviour problems are not severe, the parents should be given reassurance that the behaviour is quite normal and advice on how best to manage it. In most cases, the parents should try to remain as calm as possible and to avoid confrontation where possible. It is often best to ignore the disturbed behaviour or distract the child into some other activity. Fussing, getting angry or upset often makes the child more likely to repeat the behaviour as it is often used as a weapon to gain the parent's attention.

Reassurance and support

Some behaviours are signs of anxiety and stress and these will only get worse if the child is punished for them. For example, a school age child who is still wetting the bed should

Signs of anxiety and stress

be praised by his parents when he stays dry all night but not punished when he is wet.

Although most children encounter some psychological problems during their childhood, these are usually transient and limited in severity if the child's parents provide good role models, are warm and accepting, and are fairly consistent in their treatment of the child. If the parents need additional support and guidance, the health visitor may be willing to visit the family at home to give advice on management. When problems are severe or chronic or there is evidence of associated family difficulties, a referral to child guidance may be necessary. A clinical psychologist may be more suitable with certain behavioural disturbances, such as enuresis, which are amenable to behaviour therapy techniques.

Usually transient

Health visitor

Clinical psychologist

Child guidance service

Child guidance clinics are normally the joint responsibility of the local education authorities and the area health authorities. The clinics are staffed by a team usually including psychiatrists, educational psychologists and social workers. The setting of this service varies according to the area, in one locality the service may be based in a hospital, in another it may be based in a health centre.

Clinics have several functions but in most cases they act as treatment centres for the emotional disturbed child and will take referrals of preschool and school age children from general practitioners. The team of specialists makes a study of the child and his family, including their past history and the child's school record. Recommendations for treatment may include therapeutic work with the child and his family at the clinic, or placement in a residential setting, e.g. boarding school or hostel.

The clinics also act as an advisory service to the education department and the juvenile courts. They may assess whether children are in need of special education and advise on what would be the most appropriate treatment for delinquent behaviour.

Child guidance

Can act as treatment centres

Advisory service

Educational problems

A child must normally start school once he is 5 and continue to attend regularly until he is at least 16 years old. Arrangements

22

can be made for parents to educate their own children at home, but only where the home instructor is shown to be up to legally required minimum standards.

Problems at school If there are problems at school, parents should first contact their child's teacher or the head to try and work out some solution to the problem. However, help may be obtained from the education welfare officer who is responsible for the welfare of school age children and some schools also employ special counsellors.

The role of the EWO The education welfare officer has a number of roles and tasks. One of her main duties is to ensure school attendance but she will also investigate the home circumstances of children seen at school who look neglected, rejected or emotionally disturbed. In addition, education welfare offices are involved in a great number of practical tasks, such as arranging transport for those attending special schools and assessing the eligibility of children for free school meals etc.

Involvement of EWO The education welfare officer has such a large caseload that she usually is unable to become very closely involved with any one particular case. She may help a family financially by contacting the DHSS etc., but may have to refer a family on to other agencies such as child guidance or social services for more intensive work. EWOs are often involved in the assessment of children for special education and in preparing reports of the home circumstances of children for other agencies such as child guidance.

Non-attendance

Reason for non-attendance The reasons for non-attendance vary considerably. With the very young child, the mother may find it difficult to be separated and keep the child at home. Older children may be fearful of being bullied, or frustrated because of poor school performance, or they may feel school is of little use to them.

Special centres for persistent non-attenders Where a child is persistently absent from school, the education welfare officer will visit the family at home to assess the situation. The officer has to decide whether to be sympathetic, treating the problem by offering support, practical help or referral, or whether to try to use authority and control, threatening legal action. Some areas run special day centres for persistent non-attenders in which education is given in a less formal and more supportive way.

Normally, legal action is considered the last resort, especially

Problems in social care

Legal
action

as the case may be difficult to prove. However, it can be used as a threat, compelling parents to make sure their child attends school.

School
Attendance
Order

If the parents fail to satisfy the local education authority that the child is being properly educated, the authority may serve on the parents a School Attendance Order which will involve a juvenile court appearance. Alternatively, the child may be brought before the juvenile court by the social services department under the Children and Young Persons Act.

The juvenile court may decide on a number of options, and if the home circumstances are very poor a Care Order can be made.

Child abuse

During the last 10-15 years, there has been a great deal of concern over the number of children treated cruelly by their parents, either physically, mentally or both. There has been a number of well publicized tragedies where the professionals involved have been criticized. This has led to a considerable tightening up of professional procedures with cases of potential or actual abuse.

Children most at risk

Those
most 'at risk'

The risk that parents will hurt their children are greater when the parents are unstable people, when they live in stressful conditions and when the child is first born. Parents who have unhappy, disturbed backgrounds are more likely to harm their children. They are often emotionally immature and have no model on which to base good parenting. A long separation after the baby's birth may also be another factor. Young single mothers are also at risk or those with young immature boyfriends or husbands. A fretful grizzly baby or a disobedient toddler with trantrums will only make matters worse.

Mental
cruelty

In addition to children who are subject to physical cruelty, there are those who are persecuted mentally by one or both parents. One child of the family may be singled out for harsh treatment and receive mental and possibly physical cruelty as well. The child could have been unwanted from conception or the reason why the parents married. Alternatively,

24

he may have been a difficult baby, always crying, rarely sleeping and hard to feed.

The general practitioner needs to be alert to physical symptoms and to the child's attitude towards his parents and other adults. The child's behaviour can often reveal his parent's rejection. He may cringe, be constantly tired or ill or be overtly attention-seeking and demanding. A child with suspicious injuries should be asked how he obtained them. If there is no reasonable or ready explanation, the social services department or the National Society for Prevention of Cruelty to Children should be contacted so the situation can be investigated.

Alert to symptoms

Procedure after notification

If a suspicious incident happens or there is reason to believe that a child is being persistently neglected or cruelly treated, the social services department should be notified or the NSPCC who will send a social worker to visit the family at home. The social worker will decide whether the family needs help and whether there is cause for concern.

Notification of child to social services department

If there is any reason to suspect neglect or ill treatment, a case conference will be arranged where all the professionals concerned with the family (health visitor, social worker, doctor, teacher) will be invited to attend. Although general practitioners rarely attend these conferences, they do have an important role, often having more detailed knowledge of a family and their background than other agencies. They are also aware of the family's medical history and recent health, for example, whether the mother is depressed. It is important that the assessment of the family's circumstances is as complete as possible so that a well-informed decision is made on future action. Police, school, health and social service records may all shed light on the present situation and the family dynamics.

Case conference

Role of the doctor

The members of the case conference all help to decide on future action, although the social services representative has to make the final decision as they hold most responsibility. A 'key worker' in the case may also be appointed. This could be a social worker or health visitor.

One of a number of courses of action can be taken. Normally, separating a child from his family is considered the last resort. Studies have shown that psychological damage can result from separating child and parent even when the previous

Course of action

parenting is poor. Life in care also brings with it very many problems.

The professionals involved in the case need to weigh up the risks associated with keeping the child at home with the problems which may result from separation. If it is decided that

separation is necessary, the social services department will need to initiate care proceedings (discussed later in the chapter). In most cases, the key professional involved will work within the family to ease and rectify the situation, if at all possible. All types of practical help may be given such as a day nursery placement, financial aid or help with housing.

Cases of actual or potential child abuse need very sensitive and skilful handling as well as full co-operation between the

different professions involved. Problems, often with tragic consequences, can arise when relevant information is not shared between agencies and when communication is poor.

In an emergency

If a child needs immediate protection, a Place of Safety Order

can be taken out. Social workers, doctors and NSPCC workers can obtain this Order by applying to a magistrate. The child can then be detained in a place of safety for a period of up to 28 days. A police officer also has the power to remove a child to a place of safety under his own authority. In practice, it is probably easiest if the doctor contacts the social services department and tells them of the urgency of the situation.

Places of safety are usually in a hospital or a children's home. Before it expires, a decision has to be made to let the child return to his parents, to receive him into care on the parents' application, or bring him before a juvenile court and seek some kind of protective order. It is during this period of 4 weeks that the assessments and conference needs to take place.

Even though the Place of Safety Order is temporary, it is always a serious matter separating children from their parents and there must be a sound and reasonable ground for this action.

The need for day care

Day care can provide the mother with the opportunity to work and can give relief to other mothers who find it hard to cope.

Children and young people

Advantages of day care Many child care problems can be helped or alleviated by the provision of good day care facilities for the under fives or for school children after school hours and during the holidays. Good day care can offer a stimulating environment, free from stress. In addition, playgroups can offer all young children a range of different activities, friendship and prepare them for school.

Details from SSDS or health visitors Details of day nurseries, child-minders and playgroups in the area are available from the social services departments who have a duty to register and supervise all these facilities. Health visitors will also have personal experience regarding the facilities in their area.

Day nurseries

Day nurseries These are either run by the local authority or privately. They are open most of the year and their hours are similar to an adult's working day. Places in the local authority nurseries are usually difficult to obtain except for families in great need. They are usually heavily subsidized and charges are normally dependent on the family's income.

Avoiding reception into care A day nursery place may help a family to cope and can in some instances avoid reception into care of one or more children. Usually in an emergency, a day nursery place can be found to alleviate stress in the family. It is also an alternative to care when the mother has to enter hospital and the father can look after the children during the evening and night. An applicant should contact the social services department. Recommendation from a doctor (or health visitor, social worker) may help obtain a place.

Private facilities The number of private day nurseries varies according to the area. They tend to be expensive for families on low incomes but enable a mother to work. Increasingly, however, factories, offices and hospitals are providing creches or nurseries close to work.

Child-minders

Child-minders Social services departments have the duty of registering and supervising people who look after other people's children for longer than 2 hours a day, and for financial reward (close relatives are exempted, however). The number of child-minders available depends on the area. Where there is a high demand for female labour or where living costs are so high, there may be a big demand for child-minders. A good child-minder may be the best alternative to day care for a baby or a very young child as it provides more continuity than a nursery with several staff who may leave or go on holiday. Patients may usually obtain a list of registered child-minders from the social services department and they make arrangements with the child-minders themselves.

Nursery schools and classes

These are provided by some local education authorities for pre-school children. They are part of the educational system and keep school hours and school holidays, so may not be suitable for a mother who has to work. Nursery schools and classes run by the education authority are free and are staffed by teachers.

The local education office have details of nursery schools and admission is usually arranged by going to the school itself and seeing the headmistress, although long waiting lists are common. Some education authorities provide no nursery school education at all.

In addition to local authority provision, there are a number of private nursery schools. These also have long waiting lists so it is often advisable to apply early.

Playgroups and creches

In most areas there are a number of schemes whereby groups of children meet and play on one or more mornings or afternoons each week. Playgroups usually accept children over the age of 2½ or 3 and some will also accept a proportion of handicapped children.

In addition to playgroups, there may be a number of creches available whose main aim is to give mother and child a short break from each other. These creches may be found in sports centres, in further education establishments and in some health centres.

Day care facilities for older children

Many schools and local authorities provide play centres after school hours and in the school holidays to cater for the needs of children. This is particularly helpful to those children whose mothers are working. Details of these schemes are available from the local education authority or the library.

Other problems with child care

Some parents find great difficulties coping with their children and, although the child may not be physically or mentally ill-treated, he may be neglected or deprived of good physical and emotional care.

Children can suffer considerably when the relationship bet-ween the parents is poor. The period of stress and conflict which precedes the final breakdown of a family may be a particularly difficult period for the children. However, it is often better if the parents separate rather than live together in misery, squabbling and fighting.

The single parent, in most cases the mother, will also find difficulties in coping. One of the greatest problems is that the sons in the family have no paternal model. How a boy child will react will depend on his age when his father left and the quality of the relationship. If the relationship was poor, the child may be difficult to handle and react against all males. If the father left when his son was very young, the boy will have learnt little of the male role and what it means to be a husband or father.

Separation from parents may also be damaging to the child, affecting his emotional development. Disruptions in maternal care may be as damaging as poor care. Children who have been separated from their parents may find it difficult to socialize, show depressed or aggressive behaviour or are unable to sustain good relationships.

When parents or a parent have difficulty with child care, the health visitor or local authority social worker may be able to help by giving practical help as well as counselling. Often the mother needs someone to talk to at length about her own feelings and difficulties. When she is given support, reassurance and confidence in herself, she may in turn have more love and patience to give to her children.

Practical help, such as a day nursery placement or an introduction to a playgroup or club, may also be helpful. The social services department can give financial help in certain circumstances but only when they can show that it has prevented reception into care or a juvenile court appearance.

Marital breakdown

The single parent

Disruptions in continuity of care

Health visitor or social worker referral

Practical help

Financial
help

'Section 1' money can be used to pay off an electricity bill in order to stop disconnection or to pay off other debts. However, this financial payment is entirely discretionary and local authorities vary considerably in how much money they are willing to pay out or lend. For example, many local authorities will not pay off electricity bills but will temporarily lend a Calor Gas stove so that the family can still cook after disconnection.

Voluntary
organizations

Voluntary organizations, such as the Family Service Units and the Family Welfare Association, are often able to work intensively with families with many problems. The NSPCC and the Church of England Children's Society also run a number of preventive schemes for families in difficulties.

Reception into care by the local authority

Reception
into care

Statistics indicate that, on any particular day, approximately five out of every 1000 children under 18 will be in the care of local authority. One or both parents can apply for their child or children to be 'received into care' by approaching the the social services department. Friends or relatives left with a child can also do this. If the problem is urgent, a prompt visit by a social worker will be made to the home.

Children are received into care for a number of reasons. They may have become orphans or have been abandoned. Their parents may not be able to look after them, sometimes due to physical or mental disability.

Prevention of
reception into
care

All efforts are made, however, to avoid reception into care where possible because of the harmful effects it may have on the children involved. A number of alternatives may be suggested to keep the children at home. For example, a day nursery place and a home help may enable the father to cope when the mother is ill in hospital. Some local authorities employ special child helpers who look after the family in their own home when the mother is away temporarily.

Places of care

By whatever means a child comes into care, the duty of the local authority is to consider the welfare of the child in deciding where to place him. Children are either boarded out with foster parents, placed in a community home or a specialist establishment such as a boarding school.

In England and Wales, about half of all the children in care

Children and young people

are boarded out with foster parents. The child who is fostered will be afforded the opportunity of having a normal family life while he is in care.

In some circumstances, relatives or friends of the family may be willing to act as foster parents but cannot afford the maintenance. In these cases, if the social worker involved approves, they can be made foster parents and paid the main-tenance allowance.

Community homes

Local authorities and registered voluntary organizations also provide residential establishments for children in care called 'community homes'. The range of residential care provided by community homes varies from residential nurseries to hostels for those over compulsory school age and includes establishments where children live in 'family' groups.

Loss of parental rights

When a child is received into care voluntarily, the social worker involved must keep the parents informed of their child's welfare. During the first 6 months, parents can visit as they like and take him home when they want. After this, how-ever, parents may lose some of their rights. They have, for example, to give 28 days notice to the local authority of their intention to remove the child from care. This is to ensure that the child is prepared to return to his parents and that it is not a sudden and unexpected change.

After 6 months, the local authority can also take over parental responsibility for a child, assuming 'parental rights' over a child in their care or a Care Order can be made by the juvenile courts. When parental rights are taken over, the parents lose the freedom to visit when they want or to take the child home. However, parents can appeal against their loss of parental rights to the courts.

Reception into care against parents' wishes

Local authorities can also receive children into their care against their parents' wishes by going through the juvenile courts and obtaining a Care Order. However, local authorities are very much beset by rules and regulations and what may be considered best for the child by the professionals involved may not be legally permissible.

Care proceedings

A local authority can bring about care proceedings if it considers that a child or young person is in need of care and protection or is beyond parental control. These proceedings may also be instigated by the police, the local education authority or another agency such as the NSPCC.

Juvenile courts may make a Care Order when it has been proved that the child is in need of care and control which he is unlikely to receive unless an Order is made. In addition, one of the following conditions has to be proved: (1) that he is being ill-treated or his proper development is being prevented or his health is being neglected; (2) that he is exposed to moral danger; (3) that he is beyond the control of his parent or guardian; (4) that he is not receiving efficient full-time education suitable to his age, ability and aptitude; (5) that he is guilty of an offence.

When a Care Order is made, parents lose virtually all rights to control the child and the child must reside where the local authority directs. Although Care Orders remain in force until the child becomes 18, the local authority, parents or child can apply to the court to have the Order discharged. Instead of a

Care Order, the courts may make a Supervision Order, a Hospital or Guardianship Order under the Mental Health Act, an Interim Care Order, or make an Order requiring his parents to take proper care and control over him.

A Supervision Order places the child under the supervision of a local authority social worker or a probation officer. The supervising officer must have access to the child and can bring him back to court if necessary. These Orders may also contain directions relating to residence, medical treatment and intermediate treatment.

Problems of adolescence

Adolescence can be a particularly stressful and difficult period for both the child and his parents. It is a time when the rapid physical and physiological changes taking place may make the adolescent awkward and self-conscious about his appearance and emerging sexuality. The young person also has to cope with the difficult transition from childish dependence to adult independence and develop a sense of his own personal identity. The young adult has to prepare himself for his future life, choose a job or career, prepare for sexual maturity, decide on the goals in his life and a personal philosophy.

The ease with which the adolescent achieves a strong sense of identity and his sexual adjustment will depend very much on the nature of his previous and current relationship **Peer** with his parents. However, his relationships with his peers are **relationships** also of crucial importance. The adolescent has a great need to conform to the values and customs of others in the same age group and will sometimes accept these as his own although contrary to those of his parents. If he mixes with delinquents or drug takers, he may easily start these behaviours himself.

The 'ill at ease' adolescent who lacks self-confidence may become a social isolate who is timid, nervous and withdrawn. **Danger of** He can feel intensely lonely and depressed, especially as his **depression** relationships with his peers are all important to him. Alternatively, the adolescent may react by over compensating, becoming aggressive, attention-seeking and conceited.

The young person's conflict between his dependence on his parents and his desire for independence may result in **Rebellion** rebellion and rejection of the parents. This often occurs when **and rejection** the parents have been over protective and have allowed the child little freedom, thus causing resentment.

The doctor may find himself having to mediate between **Doctor as** parents and child. As with a marital problem, he can often help **mediator** by getting 'each side' to see the other's point of view.

In addition to the services available for younger children there are a number of advisory or counselling centres specifically for young people. These centres vary considerably **Advisory and** in the help offered, ranging from those which offer professional **counselling** advice and counselling to those staffed entirely by volunteers. **services** Some have also developed information services. Problems discussed often include those on education, work or health, as well as personal problems. The Citizens' Advice Bureau will know of the centres in the locality. The young person can usually telephone for help or in some cases call personally.

Social activities

Often young people can be kept out of trouble and can lead a more satisfying life if they belong to one of a number of

33

clubs in their area with activities geared to their age group and personal interests.

There are youth clubs in most areas and these are often organized by the churches, the local education authority or a number of voluntary organizations such as the National Association of Boys' Clubs or the YMCA. Detailed information *Youth clubs* about schemes can be obtained from the local education authority or the National Youth Bureau.

There are a number of organizations which set up projects where young volunteers help those in need in a variety of *Voluntary* different ways, such as gardening and decorating old peoples' *workers* flats. Task Force and the Young Volunteer Force operate these projects. Community service volunteers also provide full-time work on a food, bed and pocket-money basis.

Accommodation problems

Young people often have problems in obtaining suitable accommodation, especially if they leave home and move to *Accommo-* another town. The YMCA and YWCA may be able to help and *dation* they run a special accommodation advisory service in London. There are also a number of other centres offering help and accommodation in the capital.

Careers advice and unemployment

Unemployment in young school leavers can cause great distress, disillusionment, alienation and frustration. However, young people are entitled to the same services as adults for *Careers* employment advice and help. The local education authority *advice* runs a careers advice service and careers officers visit schools *service* and then make arrangements for individual interviews.

There are a number of schemes set up specifically to help unemployed young people obtain a job or train for one. Details are available at job centres, Department of Employment or at the schools.

Juvenile delinquency

A sizeable proportion of all offences are committed by young people. There is much evidence to suggest that delinquent or deviant behaviour in older children is linked with bad experiences in childhood, with deprivation and inconsistent care. However, the social conditions of the neighbourhood also affect rates of juvenile delinquency and the particular school attended. Recently, there has been an alarming increase in the amount of crime committed by girls and a greater degree of female aggressiveness.

There are a number of agencies who help the families of offenders as well as the offenders themselves. These include the local authority social services department and the probation service. If legal help is necessary, some parents on low incomes may be eligible for legal aid but others can obtain advice or help from a law centre or legal advice centre.

Most police forces now caution 50% of juvenile first offenders. The child and his parents are brought before a senior police officer who warns the child, telling him to mend his ways. In some areas, juvenile bureaux and other schemes have been set up where police officers liaise with other professionals before deciding on future action.

A child will be brought before a juvenile court if the police decide to prosecute. If the child is found guilty, the magistrates normally require reports about a child before deciding on what action to take. In some cases, the child may be remanded on bail or in custody for further reports. The magistrates have a number of options of disposal, they can give the child an absolute or conditional discharge, they can fine him or bind him over to his parents, or they can make a Supervision, Care or Attendance Centre Order. Older children may be sent to a detention centre or Borstal training (the latter only by a Crown court).

Probation service

Legal aid and advice

The use of caution

The juvenile court

Summary of services and help available

Agency	*Type of help*
Health visitors (local area health authority)	Advice, assistance and emotional support to families with a child care problem especially for the under fives

Social workers (local authority social services department)	Assistance in child care problems especially the more serious ones including:
	    child abuse (including applying for a Place of Safety Order)
	    voluntary reception into residential care
	    juvenile delinquency
	    reception into care through the juvenile courts
	    the need for day care facilities
	    fostering/adoption

Social workers can assist by providing practical help, counselling, and sometimes by giving financial aid. Social services departments also have a day-care section with details of private day-care facilities including playgroups, child-minders and private nurseries.

Child guidance (including clinical psychologists)	Advice, assistance and treatment for preschool and school age children and their families
Local education authority	Schooling and sometimes nursery school provision
	Careers advice through careers officers
	Educational welfare officers who can assist with all education difficulties including practical matters
	Additional facilities for school children after hours or in the holidays (available in some local authorities)
Department of employment (local employment offices)	Careers assistance
	Help with finding employment
	Details of courses of further training

Summary of services and help available (continued)

Probation officers (probation service)	Advice, assistance and support for the older child who is an offender
Voluntary organizations	Emotional support and counselling for families (including intensive help in some cases)
	Counselling and information services for young adults
	Financial assistance
	Day care and play facilities
	Social, leisure activities and youth clubs
	Residential provision for children
	Accommodation for young adults
	Specialized schools

4 Problems of adult and family life

Marital difficulties and divorce

Increase in divorce rate

While the number of marriages has varied little during the past 15 years, the number of divorces has risen dramatically, affecting a large number of adults and children. In 1975, for instance, 12 522 couples in England and Wales were granted a divorce which meant that 443 519 individuals were affected including children. This increase in divorce rate is due to a number of factors, such as the introduction of the Divorce Reform Act in 1969, the greater availability of legal aid and changes in the practice of financial settlements. There is also less stigma attached to being divorced and women are more able to lead independent lives.

Although divorce rates have increased, it is difficult to ascertain whether marital problems and breakdowns have shown a similar rate of increase during recent years. Divorce rates reflect only a proportion of marriages which are in trouble. Many couples with severe problems still stay together or separate without any legal action.

Predictors of failure

Cycle of deprivation

Although poverty and other material deprivation impose great strains on the marital relationship, marital difficulties are found in all social classes and income groups. There are, however, certain known predictors of marital breakdown. It is more frequent when the couple married at an early age, when they have few friends, when they have had relatively little education and when their life style is unconventional. It is a sad fact that children brought up in disturbed and unhappy families with marital strife often grow up to make unsatisfactory marriages themselves. They are often insecure and have never had adequate role models of how to be a 'good' husband and father or wife or mother. This has been called 'the cycle of deprivation'.

Personality traits

Psychological studies have also shown that certain personality traits can predict failure in marriage. If the husband is considered emotionally immature or if either partner is emotionally unstable, marital breakdown is likely. If a couple are able to communicate well, can handle conflict and show a high level of emotional support, their marriage is less likely to break down. However, it is difficult to disentangle cause and effect.

Expectations too high

The changing role of women in society must also place extra strains on marriage. Men and women often have too high expectations of marriage and discontentment arises from the gap between these high aspirations and actual experience.

Effect on health

The highest rates of breakdown occur in the first years of marriage with couples who never adjust satisfactorily to living with one another. However, breakdown is usually preceded by months or years of intense conflict affecting all family members. Women have been shown to experience many health problems related to marital stress and these are often particularly noticeable in the period prior to separation. They may be depressed or anxious and unable to cope or complain of headaches, listlessness, etc. Husbands may also become ill or start to drink excessively.

Depression and alcoholism result

These problems do not end, however, when the couple become divorced. Research with divorcees has also revealed a high degree of stress and unhappiness which may last a very long time. The status of divorce is associated with a high risk of clinical depression, alcoholism and attempted suicide. Depression may result from the lack of social support, the absence of a close and intimate relationship and a loss of self-esteem. Coping with the children alone or losing daily contact with them may also bring its problems.

Effect on children

It is the children who usually suffer the most; marital turmoil often has long-term consequences on the children's personality, behaviour and schooling. Children from broken homes have been shown to do worse at school and exhibit more maladjusted or delinquent behaviour than children who lose a parent by death. The frequent quarrels or unpleasantness between a couple when still living together can result in the children showing symptoms of anxiety and insecurity, such as loss of appetite, nail biting, bedwetting, regression or poor physical health.

The stress on the children may be alleviated when and if the parents separate unless the parents still continue their fight by trying to put their children against the other parent. Divorce or separation can mean, however, that the child will lose contact with one of his parents. One recent investigation showed that over half of the children in the study lost contact with one of their parents within a few months of the separation.

Where people go for help with marital problems

The studies conducted in this area all indicate that family doctors are the most frequently consulted professional for marital problems. One study of women who had petitioned for a divorce found that 90% had approached their doctor for help.

Often, however, the men and women attend for some other matter apparently unconnected with the marriage. Most doctors have seen patients complaining of depression, headaches, or behavioural problems in a child and although these problems are real enough, the underlying problem is an unhappy marriage. It is important for the doctor to be alert to the signals of marital disharmony and not ignore them.

Recognition of problems

There are many reasons why most men and women approach their doctor for help rather than a more specific agency. Attending a marriage guidance agency takes courage and initiative but it also means that the person involved has accepted that his marriage is in difficulty, which represents failure. People know little of what goes on in these agencies and what they will be asked to do and so may be too anxious or fearful to attend. In smaller communities, the individual may also be afraid of being seen entering the agency.

Fear of marriage guidance

Approaching the family doctor, on the other hand, is much less threatening. First, there is no stigma attached to attending. Secondly, the patient is more familiar with the surgery and the doctor concerned. He or she may have attended with other problems and been sympathetically received and helped. Even under these circumstances, however, patients may not readily admit to their marital problem or ask for help and will only do so after delicate questioning by the doctor.

Reason why doctor approached

Many doctors, when confronted with a patient with a marital problem, may react by referring the patient elsewhere. However it is important to realize that the patient has chosen the doctor as the person to which he wishes to divulge his problem. The patient may regard a speedy referral to another

The dangers associated with immediate referral

41

agency as a personal rejection. If he was too fearful to attend another agency in the first place, he may still refuse to go and may keep his problems to himself in future. Often, patients will need help, advice and support from their doctor before they are able to seek help from elsewhere.

Offering support and advice

The doctor can often help considerably by listening, offering sympathy, advice and guidance. Dealing with marital problems, however, needs a certain degree of confidence in tackling such sensitive issues. Often, personal anxieties about one's own marriage can be involved.

Joint interviewing

More progress can often be made if the couple are seen together and the difficulties of the relationship are seen from both points of view. Problems often arise through poor communication between partners and often greater understanding can result from an interview where the doctor is an intermediary. Alternatively, the doctor can attempt to alter the behaviour of each spouse. He can, for example, draw up a list for husband and wife of the behaviours which are disliked and liked by the spouse. The couple can then agree on some plan for a specific period whereby they reduce the 'disliked' behaviours and increase the 'liked' ones.

Behaviour changes

Focus on the couple

Whether the doctor sees one patient individually or the couple, his focus should be on the couple and their relationship rather than the individual. Resistance to change is usually encountered, however, even in those who want to change their relationship. People usually experience emotional pressures within themselves to maintain the status quo. Change is usually difficult as it means that the person has to give up the established way he has built up to protect himself from anxiety and distress.

When couples decide to separate, help is still necessary as each will need to adjust to a life apart and to cope with the feelings incurred such as anger, depression or resentment.

Specific counselling agencies for marriage

Referral to a counselling service may be helpful if the couple are willing and ready. There are a number of agencies who can help.

Marriage guidance councils

There are 150 local marriage guidance councils in England, Wales and Northern Ireland and there is a service in Scotland

Marriage guidance

as well. Although some of their work is involved in educating and preparing for marriage, marriage guidance counsellors also work with individuals and couples with marital problems. They usually work intensively and in depth. Although they prefer to see both husband and wife, they will take on cases where only one of the couple will attend.

Counsellors are unpaid but have to go through a rigorous selection procedure before they are accepted for training. Counsellors attend a residential basic training course, a subsequent in-service training course and regular supervision. The services are open to couples of all religions.

In recent years, schemes have been set up whereby marriage guidance counsellors are attached to general practices, taking referrals directly from the doctors involved and sometimes seeing patients in the surgery. These schemes can be very successful and approximately 100 of them are now in operation.

Other marriage guidance councils

Other councils

The Catholic Marriage Guidance Council also relies on volunteers and is available to Catholics with marital difficulties. Jews can receive help from the Jewish Marriage Education Council or the Jewish Welfare Board.

Probation officers and social workers

The role of the probation officer

One of the roles of probation officers involves attempting conciliation before a divorce or separation. Probation officers are also obliged to make a report on the custody or welfare of a child in a divorce case when requested by the court. From these statutory duties, there has grown the practice of giving help to those with marital problems when the court is not involved and probation officers have become known as the professional to whom these types of problems can be taken. Social workers can also undertake marital therapy and this can be a major part of their work with problem families.

Other voluntary agencies

In addition to these agencies, the Family Welfare Association, a voluntary organization, specializes in giving help to families in distress. A major part of their work is marital therapy whereby couples are given counselling help.

43

Battered wives

This problem is found in families of all social classes. It may occur with husbands who are generally caring and responsible and whose outbursts are therefore out of character. Excessive drinking, stress or jealousy may be the cause of the violence. It is sometimes difficult for the wife to admit to having been beaten. She may attempt to conceal the bruises or give another explanation.

Wives may find the violence leaves them bewildered and uncertain of whether to separate from their husband, especially if he vows never to do it again. In many cases, the women have nowhere to go to and it is for this reason that a number of refuges have been set up specifically for battered wives. They offer temporary accommodation for women and their children who have suffered physical violence or mental suffering. A number of voluntary groups also offer advice and support to women in need of help (see appendices). A woman can also apply to court to take out an injunction forbidding her husband to return to the family home.

Refuges for battered wives

Separation

Separation

Legal separation may be brought about either by mutual agreement or by a Court Order. Financial help is available under legal aid schemes and it is advisable before taking action in a court to consult a solicitor or probation officer.

Those who wish to go to court can apply to the magistrates court. Normally, a probation officer will visit to investigate whether reconciliation is possible.

Divorce

Grounds for divorce

Under the Divorce Reform Act, 1969, the only grounds for divorce are that the marriage has irretrievably broken down. Adultery, cruelty or desertion may be used as evidence, however. A divorce may be granted when a couple both agree that they want to end their marriage and have been separated for 2 years. If one partner objects, it is necessary to have been separated for 5 years.

Appearance in court

For an uncomplicated divorce (where both partners are in agreement over property and custody of children) the couple do not need to appear in court. Legal aid can be granted for other types of divorce but not for undefended divorce. It is possible to get a divorce without the help of a solicitor and details can be obtained from the divorce court office or the Citizens' Advice Bureau.

Help with sexual problems

Unsatisfactory sexual relationships can give rise to a number of psychological and physiological disorders. They can also lead to an unhappy marriage, infidelity or divorce.

A person's sexuality is an interaction between emotional attitudes and physical performance. However, great anxieties about failure and inadequacy are often associated with sexual performance. Sexual problems may be physically based, or *Origin of* due to difficulties in communication between partners or due *sexual* to conflicts within an individual or within a relationship. *problems* There is also a great variation between individuals in their sexual needs and problems can occur when there is a great discrepancy between partners.

As with marital problems, the doctor must decide whether he should handle the problem himself or refer to another agency. If he decides to refer to another agency, he should do this when the individual or couple is ready, as an immediate referral may be regarded as a rejection.

Treatment of sexual problems may involve, solely or in combination, psychoanalytical techniques, counselling, marital therapy, behaviour therapy, advice and the use of drugs or other aids. The doctor may aid communication between a couple by asking them both to attend to discuss their problems or difficulties. Problems in discrepancy in needs between partners can be helped by getting each individual to agree to a 'happy medium' between them and to be more toler- ant of each other's desires. Behaviour therapy has been used *Behaviour* increasingly with sexual problems and a variety of counsellors *therapy* are now trained to use these therapeutic techniques, including some marriage guidance counsellors.

Agencies who can help

There are a number of National Health Service clinics which are involved in the treatment of sexual problems. They may be part of the psychiatric, obstetric and gynaecology departments

45

Other agencies involved

and the staff involved are likely to be psychiatrists, psychologists, social workers or nurses. These clinics use a variety of treatment ranging from brief psychotherapy and behavioural techniques to marital therapy.

Marriage guidance counsellors may also be able to help if the sexual difficulty is based on a marital problem. Some family planning clinics also run psychosexual counselling services (details from the Family Planning Association).

One-parent families

Extent of problem

Children are raised in single-parent families when the mother has not married, when there has been a divorce or separation, or when one parent has died. In 1971, there were reckoned to be 620 000 one-parent families in Great Britain, of which 100 000 were motherless and the rest fatherless. Nearly one tenth of all families with dependent children have one parent.

Hardships

One-parent families face many hardships. The children have many emotional problems which affect all aspects of their life including their health. Even after the separation, the parents may still fight over access using the children as pawns in the battle.

Isolation

Whether divorced, separated, widowed or unmarried the single-handed mother or father has a number of problems. He or she may be lonely or socially isolated with no one to give the emotional support and adult company so necessary when bringing up a family. The single-handed parent also has to try and meet the emotional needs of the children and take on the traditional roles of the other parent as well.

Absence of mother

When the father is absent (as in the majority of cases) the boys in the family have no paternal model to imitate. However, a father left with young children may face even greater difficulties than the mother. He may be unused to doing all the domestic duties and chores. He will also be subjected to a number of other pressures deterring him from looking after the family itself. Other male friends may regard his changed role as 'being sissy'. He will also find it difficult to make friends he can visit in the daytime as women at home with their children may view him with suspicion. The father living on social security may also find he is under some pressure from the DHSS to go back to work.

46

Problems of adult and family life

Financial problems

Single-parent families are often on the poverty line or suffer some degree of financial hardship. The homes of single-parent families are often overcrowded and lacking in basic amenities. Those who choose not to work are eligible for supplementary benefit if their income or savings are not too high. A slightly higher rate is paid if on long-term benefit. Child benefit is also paid at a higher rate.

Increased benefits and allowances

The single parent who decides to work has a higher tax allowance. They also may be eligible for family income supplement. However, many single parents do not find it worth while to work as they have to pay out a large proportion of their income for daytime care of their children.

Loneliness and isolation

The single parent is less likely to be able to organize a social life and finding a babysitter can be a problem. During times of parental illness, there may be few additional social resources to call upon. There are now a number of self-help groups for single parents covering most areas. As with other self-help groups, parents can share their problems and help each other, giving support and friendship. The National Council for One Parent Families may also be able to help. It has a welfare department and employs social workers. They give advice on practical, housing, financial and legal problems.

Voluntary organizations

The unmarried mother

The unmarried expectant mother may find it hard to admit to her pregnancy and faces many problems once she does so. The local authority social services department should be notified of any pregnancy when the girl is under 17.

Notification of pregnant girls under 17

The unmarried mother will have to make an early decision about whether she should seek a termination of her pregnancy, whether she should keep the child or have it adopted. She will need help and support in making this decision, especially if the parents and boyfriend do not know or are unhelpful.

There are a number of agencies to help the unmarried mother before and after her pregnancy. These include health visitors, hospital and local authority social workers, adoption agencies, organizations run by religious bodies and those for

Agencies who can help

47

single-parent families. Some of the voluntary organizations run by the churches are able to carry out intensive work.

Accommoda-
tion problems

These agencies can help find the mother a place to stay before and after the birth in a hostel or mother and baby home. Accommodation may be difficult to obtain after this period although homeless single-parent families are eligible for council accommodation.

Affiliation
Orders

For the child, there are still some legal disadvantages in being born illegitimate but there are plans to reduce these in the future. The mother can try to get financial help from the father of the child by applying to court for an Affiliation Order. If the parents do eventually marry, the child becomes legitimate and the parents can apply for the re-registration of the child's birth. If the mother marries someone other than the child's father, the couple can apply to adopt the child.

The unmarried mother is eligible for supplementary benefit or family income supplement if she is at work on a low income. She may also be eligible for maternity allowances.

Multi-problem families

Most general practitioners will have amongst their patients a number of families who lurch from one crisis to another. The parents may be below average in intelligence, they may have low incomes or be living on benefits. They may be unable to budget wisely and thus build up debts and rent arrears and are unable to pay their fuel bills. In addition, the parents may be unhappily married and the children neglected.

These families impose great strains on all those who try to help them. They take up an inordinate amount of time as well as patience. Health visitors or social workers (often both) may also be involved. Sometimes, intensive social work involvement may help. A number of voluntary organizations specialize in helping these families (Family Service Units or the Family Welfare Association). Details of these agencies are available from their head offices or the Citizens' Advice Bureau.

Bereavement and widowhood

There are a number of commonly observed characteristics of grief: shock, denial, anxiety, depression, guilt, anger and a

Character-
istics of grief
wide variety of somatic signs of anxiety. Other components include suicidal thoughts, searching behaviour, idealization of the lost person and panic. Losing a spouse can result in a raised general death rate, an increased suicide rate as well as increased rates of consultations with general practitioners and psychiatrists.

Many observers consider there are a number of stages to mourning, namely, shock, despair and recovery. However, people do not always progress from one stage to another in an orderly sequence, the stages merge and overlap with frequent regressions.

The initial
shock
Initially, there may be a period of numbness and detachment; the person may be outwardly calm or completely dazed and disorganized. The person may at first deny the death has occurred.

The period of
acute distress
As awareness of the loss develops, the person may express anger at himself or others (including the medical profession) for not preventing the death. He may also feel guilty or wish to find a scapegoat. During this period of 'painful pining', the bereaved person will feel intense feelings of grief, accompanied by much somatic distress. He may be restless and preoccupied with thoughts of the lost person, including having vivid nightmares and hallucinations of the deceased. People may become frightened by the intensity of their emotions and will need reassurance that they are not going mad and that their feelings are a natural response. Talking and thinking about the deceased will usually exacerbate the distress but it is important that the bereaved person can express his feelings openly and does not try to conceal them. This acute despair phase typically lasts from 3 to 10 weeks but can take longer.

Reconstr-
uction
The final stage is the long process of recovery and recon- struction. When it is the spouse that has died the survivor has to develop new roles, new behaviours and new relationships with others. During this stage, there is a reduction in the frequency and intensity of the periods of distress and the person may start to think and attend to other things. This period of adjustment may never be complete but usually takes from 6 to 18 months.

Determinants
of the inten-
sity of grief
The degree of grief is likely to be increased when the bereavement occurs as one of a series of life crises, when the death is sudden, unanticipated and untimely (i.e. when the deceased is young or a child), when the relationship with the deceased person was very close or ambivalent and when the survivor was heavily reliant on the deceased. Severe emotional

problems after a bereavement are more likely to occur if the person has had previous episodes of depression or finds difficulty in expressing emotions. The wife who is aware that her husband may die and has prepared practically and psychologically for the death beforehand is in a far better position to cope with the bereavement than when the death is unexpected. A very long illness, however, may increase the stress and exhaustion of the survivor and therefore increase the likelihood of an adverse reaction.

Adverse reactions

Absence of grief, episodes of panic, lasting physical symptoms, excessive guilt feelings, excessive anger or intense grief over a long period are signs of adverse grief reactions. In these cases, referral to a psychiatrist may be necessary, especially if there is a risk of suicide.

Death in a child

There are also indications of a high incidence of psychological difficulties in family members if a child in the family dies. If the death is due to a terminal illness, the parents and others usually begin to grieve soon after they accept the prognosis. Since the parents and siblings are likely to be the child's greatest source of comfort, it is important that help and support is given to them for the sake of the child's welfare as well as their own. Siblings may be profoundly affected by the illness and death of a brother or sister and exhibit behaviour disturbances or depression. Parents have to cope not only with their own grief but they have to give comfort to their other children as well as reassure the one who is ill.

Siblings also need help

Emotional support

Bereaved people do appreciate the expressions of sympathy paid to them by others. Often a squeeze of the hand or a hand on the shoulder can convey more sympathy than speech.

The need to talk

The bereaved will also need someone to whom they can talk and express their feelings. This person should not try to push them into things before they are ready, but support them emotionally and practically where appropriate. Informal support from close friends is therefore of great importance and those with religious faith may also receive help from their church. However, many people do not have many close friends or people to whom they can readily talk. In these cases it may be advisable to refer the bereaved person to a club or organization in the area whose specific aim is to help the bereaved. Cruse clubs introduce widows to each other so that they can

Informal help

Clergy

Cruse clubs and the Samaritans

meet for company, support and self-help. This organization offers a range of help from practical advice and social activities to professional counselling. Many of the bereaved also make use of the 24-hour service run by the Samaritans. The volunteers in this organization are always willing to listen to those who need to talk.

Financial hardship

Money difficulties are very common, especially among widows or when there are dependent children. The more fortunate widows benefit from the savings, investment or insurance schemes paid for by their husband. Others must rely on national insurance allowances plus, for some, their own earnings. Widows may also claim supplementary benefit if eligible. They may also be eligible to receive help from a number of voluntary organizations, especially those associated with their husband's job.

Adoption

The number of children adopted each year is falling sharply. This is due in part to the fall in birth-rate, and in the wider use of contraception and abortions. The unmarried mother who keeps her child is also given more support than before and experiences less stigma. This means that there are many more couples who wish to adopt than children available. Very few babies are offered for adoption and couples may have to consider an older child, one of mixed race or one with a degree of physical or mental handicap.

Fewer babies and children available

Of the thousands of Adoption Orders granted each year, many are made in respect of children who are in the care of one of their natural parents who has remarried. A divorced mother who has been granted custody of her children may remarry and wish to integrate her children fully into the 'new' family. In order to protect their rights of inheritance, the children have to be adopted legally.

Any child under 18 who is unmarried may be adopted. It is always necessary to try and obtain the agreement of the child's natural parents or guardians before an Adoption Order is made. The need for agreement can be overruled if the court considers there are sufficient grounds to do so. If a baby is to be

51

adopted, the natural parent can only agree to this after the baby is 6 weeks old, although the adopters can look after the baby before this.

Prospective adopters

Adopting a child requires very serious consideration. The parents need to thoroughly think through all the implications of taking on a lifetime commitment. The adopted child may be of a different colour, have some degree of handicap or may have

Problems with adopting

had a very disturbed and unhappy infancy. The older child may test his 'new' parents out and exhibit disturbed behaviours or withdraw into his shell. He may inherit certain characteristics of his parents, including health difficulties, which may make child rearing difficult.

Although a single person can adopt a child legally, this only happens rarely. Adoption agencies usually accept married couples in a certain age range.

Adoption agencies

Adoption agencies

Most local authorities (the social services department) and a number of voluntary agencies arrange adoptions. The Association of British Adoption and Fostering agencies publishes a booklet listing details of all the adoption agencies. Some organizations specialize in more 'hard to place' children.

Voluntary societies make their own conditions for would-be adopters such as religion, ages of parents, etc. Alternatively, personal arrangements can be made between the natural parents and would-be adopters or with someone else as a go between.

Social investigations

After an application is made, would-be adopters are thoroughly investigated by the agency, usually by a social worker making several home visits. The social worker will enquire into all aspects of a couple's life, the strength of their marriage, their adaptability, their own background and childhood. Medical examinations are also necessary. The adoption agencies consider that the child's needs are paramount and may, therefore, place children into families with children rather than childless parents.

Those who are 'accepted' by the agency are placed on a waiting list and they may have to wait several months or years before a particular child is suggested.

Adoption arrangements

Trial period

Adoption Orders are made through juvenile, county or high courts. A formal application to adopt is made to the court by completing a number of forms. Three months must lapse before the judge or magistrates hear and determine the case and, during this time, the child must live with his would-be adopters. After an application is made, the court appoints an officer, the guardian *ad litem*, to make the fullest possible enquiry into all aspects of the case, acting on behalf of the child.

In this 3 month period, the adopters or natural parents can change their minds. When the hearing is held, the court will be informed of the assessment of the guardian *ad litem* so that they can make a decision. The court can refuse to grant an Adoption Order and can make a temporary Interim Order instead for a probationary period. Alternatively, they can decide on a 'custodianship' Order.

Failed
adoptions

The majority of adoptions work well and provide the most satisfactory form of alternative care when the natural family has failed. Many, however, go wrong and either fail completely or the child and parents have many difficulties. Many of the children seen at child guidance or attending special schools are adopted.

It is often wise if the adopter shares all he knows about the child's background with the child. This will reduce some of the child's feelings of insecurity and bewilderment.

Access to birth records

Access to
original
birth
certificate

Once adopted, a child is re-registered on the Adopted Children's Register but the names of the natural parents are not included. However, the Children Act passed in 1975 gives an adopted person over 18 the right to obtain a copy of his or her original birth certificate. He can do this by writing to the General Register Office. For those adopted before November 1975, this process involves being interviewed by a counsellor or social worker.

Custodianship

Alternatives
to adoption

It is possible for relatives (other than parents) and others such as long-term foster parents to obtain legal custody. The

53

relatives can be given a 'custodianship' Order by the courts which gives them most of the rights and duties of a parent.

Fostering

Anyone who wishes to foster a child should apply to the social services department. They will be visited a number of times by a social worker to assess their suitability. There are, however, many difficulties involved in fostering and families need to be very stable in order to withstand the extra stresses and strains imposed. The parents' own children also have to be willing to share their mum and dad with others. The children are often very distressed at leaving home, sometimes under unpleasant circumstances and may react by either withdrawing into themselves or by being aggressive or getting into trouble with the police. The foster parent also has to cope with visits from the child's natural parents and the effects these have on the child. In addition, long-term foster parents may experience a deep sense of loss when the child returns home.

Foster parents are supervised by the social worker from the social services department who is available to give help, support and advice. However, foster parents often find the support given is less than adequate, and they have to cope mostly on their own.

Payment to foster parents in care varies from area to area. Payments are usually meant to cover the child's maintenance and not more. However, foster parents are often paid higher sums of money for difficult-to-place children.

Anyone privately fostering a child who is not related must notify the local authority unless the arrangement is very temporary, such as a holiday. Social workers have to supervise these private arrangements so that they can satisfy themselves that the child is properly looked after.

Other problems of adult life
Loneliness and isolation

There are a number of clubs to cater for adults who are lonely or isolated. As well as specialist activity and sporting clubs there are clubs for single people, single parents, widows, etc. Isolated young mothers may be put into contact with others through the health visitor. Further education courses can also be helpful in making friendships.

Marginal notes: Problems with fostering · Supervision from the SSD · Payment · Private fostering · Loneliness

54

Adult illiteracy

Illiteracy   Although very few people are completely illiterate, an estimated two million people lack the basic literacy skills. These
people will often go to great lengths to conceal their illiteracy,
although it is a considerable hindrance to their everyday life.

Tuition can be given on a one-to-one basis or by attending a
course. Details about the schemes available can be obtained
from the local library.

Other diffi-   There are many other difficulties which occur in adult life
culties   such as those associated with homosexuality, the problems of
ex-offenders, etc. Agencies available to help people with these
problems are included in the Appendices.

Summary of services and help available

Details of help for housing, financial, employment and legal
problems are included in later chapters.

Agency	Type of help
Social workers (local authority social services department)	Practical help and counselling to families and adults with a variety of problems including single parent families, battered wives, and those with marital problems
	Help for unmarried mothers including accommodation
	Help in adoption and fostering cases
Local education office	Educational and recreational classes for adults (day and evenings)
	Literacy schemes for those unable to read
Probation officers (probation office)	Emotional support and counselling for those with marital difficulties
	Help to ex-offenders and those on parole or probation

Summary of services and help available (continued)

Voluntary organizations	Help with marital and sexual problems
	Refuges and emotional support for battered wives
	Social and leisure activities for the single, married and the single parent
	Legal advice on separation and divorce
	Help to the bereaved and counselling
	Adoption/fostering services
	Help for ex-offenders
The Churches	Emotional support to all groups including the bereaved
	A social work service for unmarried mothers with a wide range of help

The elderly

The elderly

In developed countries such as the United Kingdom, there is a change in the structure of the population so that there is an increasing proportion of elderly people within the overall total. This is due to men and women living longer as well as the fall in birth-rate. The elderly in the United Kingdom, for example, have almost quadrupled in number since the beginning of the century. In 1907, they represented 6% of the population; by 1977, this figure had grown to 17%. However, future project-

Population changes

ions suggest that the proportion of the elderly in the population will remain the same as today. The most striking change in the future will be the rise in the number of people over 75 and the decline in the young elderly until the end of the century when numbers will stabilize (see Figure 1).

Social changes

Family is main provider

The family is still the main provider of community care for the elderly. Most elderly people have frequent contact with relatives, particularly their own children. Brothers, sisters, nieces and nephews can take the place of children and grandchildren when someone is childless or has lost their children.

However, surveys have shown that the availability of relatives has diminished in recent years. Nearly 30% of old people live alone and this percentage increases with age. Fewer old people see their relatives frequently. This is related to the

Availability of relatives   decline in the size of households and fewer extended families. There are fewer unmarried women who remain at home to look after their parents and fewer married women not at work. Thus, there are fewer potential carers. In addition, family ties are affected by increased mobility.

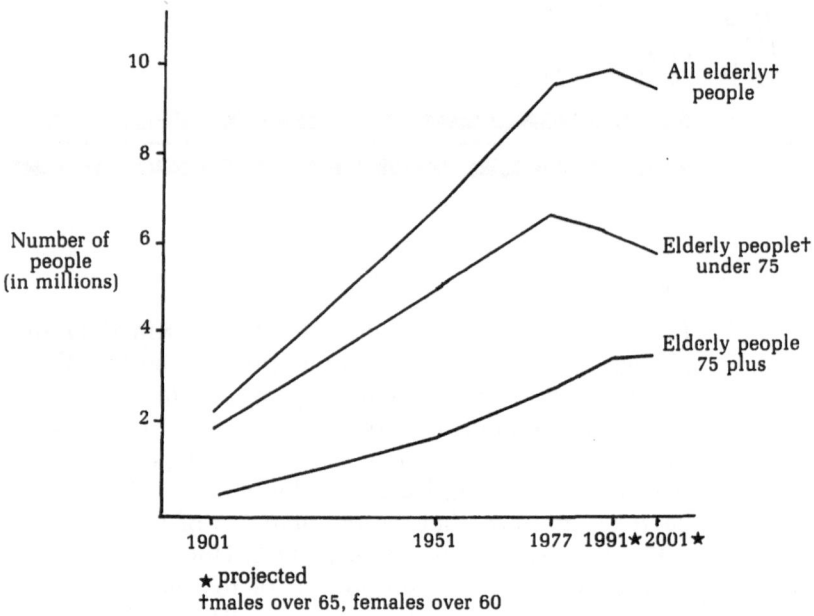

Number of people (in millions)

All elderly† people

Elderly people† under 75

Elderly people 75 plus

1901   1951   1977 1991★2001★

★ projected
†males over 65, females over 60

Figure 1   The numbers of elderly in the United Kingdom (1901–2001)

However, the general picture of old people in the United Kingdom is not too discouraging. A survey conducted in 1978 found that most people between the ages of 65 and 74 were able to go out without assistance, were basically in reasonable health and enjoyed hobbies, interests and social contacts. It is

Decline in standards with age

75+ age group most at risk   in the 75–84 age group that a moderate decline is found in mobility, health and the ability to perform personal and domestic tasks. In other things, there is a much sharper decline, as for instance in social contacts outside the home and in having hobbies and interests. Housing and financial problems are also greater. Over 85, there is an even greater decline

58

in health, social contacts and living conditions. Thus the 75+ age group, which is increasing rapidly, is the most at risk.

General services provided

Although the majority of people, who have crossed the official line to old age (over 60 for women, over 65 for men), live in reasonably good health and live active lives, they are prone to a number of social and psychological problems as well as those concerning their health. This is reflected in their use of the social and health services. Old people see their family doctors about twice as often as younger people and require more home visits. About half the patients admitted to the general wards of hospitals are over 60. Social services are also heavily used by the elderly; over three quarters of the home help force is used by people over 65 and most of those given financial help by the supplementary benefits commission are old people.

The needs of the elderly have traditionally been the concern of central and local government and of voluntary agencies. However, the division of responsibility for services between the National Health Services and the local authority (mostly the social services department) has brought many problems.

Heavy use of services

Services provided by the local authority

Local authorities are empowered to provide a number of services especially for the elderly who need help coping with daily life. In practice, there is a considerable overlap between these services and those provided for the physically handicapped. Much of their aim is to help the elderly remain comfortably in their own homes and avoid the need for residential care.

Community based services

These include a range of practical help such as the provision of home helps, meals-on-wheels and aids and adaptations to the home. Recreational and social activities may also be provided such as luncheon and social clubs, organized outings and holidays as well as transport to these facilities. The local authority also provides a social work service for advice, practical help and emotional support.

Domestic and recreational facilities

59

Residential services

Residential homes

The local authority also provides residential accommodation (old peoples' homes) for those who are unable to live at home. However, most local authorities have a number of alternative facilities such as sheltered housing with a resident warden or schemes whereby old people are boarded out in families or with landladies.

In practice, local authorities vary considerably in the services provided. Some have a wide range of facilities while others have only a few.

Voluntary organizations

Voluntary organizations

In almost all areas, there are old people's welfare associations and, in practice, the social services departments rely heavily on the contributions of local and national voluntary organizations for the elderly.

Voluntary provisions for the elderly have embraced housing, residential homes, hospitals, and many other kinds of services These are listed in the appendices.

Volunteers

Volunteers

These are often provided by a voluntary organization or by the local authority social services department. They can provide friendship for the elderly and perform simple tasks such as shopping. They can help with the decorating, gardening, cooking and doing the repairs. Personal contact has been found to be particularly valuable for the elderly, especially if unhurried.

Formal neighbourhood schemes

Good neighbours

Neighbourhood care schemes on some sort of organized basis have been in existence for many years, often under the auspices of a church. In recent years, many good neighbour schemes have been set up, sometimes based in general practice premises.

In these schemes, neighbours can shop, chat, cook, do repairs and garden. Details of any schemes in operation will be available from the social services department.

Specific problems
Psychological and social problems

Psychological
adjustment to
old age

Adjustments are necessary for people as they grow older and face a physical decline and a reduction in attractiveness. Old age brings about worries regarding health, dying and widowhood, loneliness and isolation. It may increase marital difficulties and bring about sexual problems. Old people may fear becoming dependent and having to rely on others for help; these problems may bring about withdrawal, depression and physical neglect of themselves and their homes. Specific problems will be considered in turn.

Retirement

Retirement

In recent years, fewer elderly people continue to work after the official retirement age. There are less opportunities for employment and the common stereotypes about ageing influence the behaviour of people in the employment market. These beliefs can affect recruitment, transfer, training and redundancy policies.

The man who retires at 65 can expect approximately 12 years of retirement, the woman at 60 can expect 20 years. Studies of elderly people show clearly that they are ill-prepared to cope with this proportion of their lives.

Adjusting to
retirement

Retirement brings about many difficulties in psychological and social adjustment. Work provides interest, companionship, occupation through the day, and status. The retired person has to adjust to a new life style with much more free time and a lack of a definite role in society. There is usually a reduction of income bringing about financial hardship. The problems of retirement may be greater for the manual worker who reaches the summit of his working life early. Professional people do not reach their maximum working capacity until later and after retirement can still keep an interest in their work.

Preparation for retirement

Courses on
retirement

It seems sensible, therefore, to prepare for retirement so that the individual can adjust to its limitations and benefit from its advantages. Many local authorities arrange evening or day courses on preparation for retirement. Subjects covered in these courses include living on lower incomes, health and diet, hobbies and leisure and adjusting to retirement. Details of these courses can be obtained from the local education authority or library, the Pre-Retirement Association or any local voluntary organization for the elderly. In addition, some firms organize courses for their employees.

The doctor can also encourage the retired person to use his time constructively, to act as a volunteer helper or to take up new hobbies and interests.

Loneliness and social isolation

Studies of social isolation have shown that approximately one fifth of the elderly could be considered to be isolated or extremely isolated. The elderly also consider loneliness to be their greatest problem after ill health. With the increase of elderly living alone, this problem is likely to get worse.

It must be remembered that social isolation and loneliness are not synonymous. There are two main factors in loneliness, the lack of a close relationship with another person and the emotional trauma caused by the death of one's spouse. Thus, a person surrounded by family and friends may suffer acutely from loneliness and his needs should not be overlooked.

Differences between terms

Old people may benefit by attending a social luncheon club in the area (details from the social services department). For those unable to get out, a voluntary worker may be able to visit to provide company. Voluntary organizations and good neighbour schemes can be approached to arrange such help.

Volunteers

Hobbies and interests

Many of the elderly feel unwanted and consider that they have no place in the life of the community. Having 'something to do' is one of the main prerequisites for mental health, keeping the elderly person more self-reliant and independent. Thus, the taking up of new pursuits, hobbies and learning should be encouraged.

The importance of keeping busy

Surveys have shown, however, that there is a marked fall off in interests and activities with age, especially in those confined to the house. The occupational therapist can be of help to those unable to go out but there are usually a number of opportunities available for those who have some mobility and transport can

Occupational therapist

be arranged. In addition to the special clubs in the area for the elderly (luncheon and social clubs) there are usually other recreational activities open to all age groups. Many elderly do not wish to attend functions specifically for the old and it is often better if they attend a club or a day class related to their particular interests. This will have the advantage of bringing people together because of common interests rather than age. The local education authority, library or old people's welfare organization will have details of what is provided in the area. Voluntary organizations or the social services department may be able to help with transport.

It is often forgotten that the elderly have strong desire to contribute towards the life of the community and want to feel needed and useful. They can offer a wide range of help, such as babysitting or looking after young children. Self-help groups may also be helpful. People respond more readily to the example and initiatives of their own generation.

Marginal notes: Social and luncheon clubs; Adult education courses; Transport; The need to contribute

Problems in relationships with others

Close kinship relationships can be of great value but they can also be limiting, confining and frustrating. It cannot be assumed that an elderly person living with relatives is both adequately cared for and does not suffer from loneliness.

Very close links with relatives need not always be desirable and there can be a great deal of trouble when different generations live under the same roof. This seems to happen most often when an elderly mother is living with her son and daughter-in-law and when there is friction between the women over household matters. Harmony may only be preserved if responsibilities are carefully defined and kept to. The elderly person should be allowed to reciprocate help by babysitting or looking after the children.

In some cases, a loosening of ties may constitute a desirable improvement with the elderly person either living in a granny annexe in the house doing his or her own cooking or living a short distance away. This may prevent a crisis occurring with a complete breakdown in the family relationships.

Marginal notes: Definition of responsibilities; Loosening of of ties may be desirable

The need to support the family

There are many more elderly maintained in their own homes which puts much more burden on their relatives. Thus,

Emotional and practical help

practical relief and emotional support should be provided to aged spouses, daughters and others caring for the elderly, especially when the old person is severely disabled, physically or mentally.

The strain of caring can bring about illness in the carer. Their ability to cope must be assessed and their needs recognized, thus preventing sudden breakdown in the arrangements made. There may also be an unequal distribution of caring among the different children of the family leading to anger and resentment.

Ability to cope

One of the more important services which can be provided by the local authority social services department is the provision of short-term care for the old person in an old people's home or a holiday home so that families can take a rest or a holiday. Arrangements can be made so that old people can spend regular periods away. Alternatively, old people can spend periods in hospitals if severely disabled or attend day hospitals. Extra nursing help and incontinence services should be given to families willing to care for a disabled member.

Short-term care

Day hospitals

Problems managing at home – domiciliary care

When a person needs care of some kind, this can be given in his own home, in welfare accommodation or in hospital. The place in which it is most appropriate depends on the balance between medical and social needs and whether these can be provided in the home. Many elderly people and couples live on their own without relatives because they still wish to remain independent. This desire for independence should be acknowledged and respected by any professional involved with the patient and taken into account when alternative forms of care are being considered. Since the Second World War, it has been consistent government policy to enable the elderly to continue living at home for as long as possible. To this end, legislation has been passed to enable the local authority to provide supportive services.

The desire for independence

Home help

Over half a million elderly people received assistance from the home help service in the year 1975–76. This service enables

The elderly

Home help an old person to receive domestic help for 2–3 hours per day for any number of days in the week. The duties include cleaning and tidying but may also include cooking, washing clothes and shopping. The home help may also provide the old person with much needed company and she can be used to check whether the person is becoming ill or neglecting himself.

Financial arrangements The financial arrangements vary from place to place, some authorities provide a free service, others charge according to a means test.

Meals-on-wheels

Meals-on-wheels The old person is provided with a hot midday meal on one or more days of the week which is delivered to his/her home. The old person normally pays a subsidized price. In some areas, a 7 day service is provided and emergency meals-on-wheels are available.

Luncheon clubs

Lunches In these clubs, luncheons are provided to old people who are sufficiently mobile to attend. These are preferable to meals-on-wheels as they enable the old person to get out of the house and meet others. The club supervisor can also keep a watchful eye on the state and condition of the old people who attend.

Day centres/day care

Day centres These can be predominantly social in nature or work orientated. In the former, social activities, hobbies and games are provided. In the latter, the day centre is a form of a workshop where old people can perform simple jobs and earn a little money. Transport to these clubs is often arranged through the local authority or voluntary organizations.

Day care Alternatively, a residential home or day hospital may provide day care. This type of care is useful in providing an intermediate stage between residential accommodation and staying at home.

Telephones, alarm systems and aids

Only a third of elderly people have their own telephone. However, many local authorities supply telephones to elderly

Telephones people under the Chronically Sick and Disabled Persons Act 1970. This enables the elderly person to contact relatives or professionals in an emergency. Some local authorities also provide alarm systems to alert others in an emergency. These range from buzzers and bells which alert a neighbour, to signs which can be put in a window.

Aids and adaptations Aids, appliances and adaptations to houses can also be provided by the social services department. Further details are in Chapter 6 on physical handicap.

Holidays

Holidays Local authorities sometimes organize holidays for elderly people either in their own residential homes or in ordinary holiday accommodation. In some schemes, the organization and accommodation are provided by voluntary bodies while the social services selects the individuals and pays all or part of the cost.

Problems managing at home – residential care

Part 3 accommo-dation Only a minority of old people (approximately 3%) live in residential care, and most of these are over 80 years old. Part 3 of the National Assistance Act of 1948 requires local authorities to provide residential care for elderly, which explain why the term for this type of care is often called 'Part 3 accommodation'.

Some voluntary organizations, housing associations and almshouses provide homes but the bulk of the accommodation is provided by the local authority. The local authority may use these voluntary homes and pay full or part costs. Alternatively, private homes are run where the patient or his family pay full costs.

Criteria for admission Permanent residential care is now provided by the local authority only when a person cannot manage on his own in the community even with domiciliary support and where hospital care is not needed. In general, the type of person admitted to this sort of accommodation should be reasonably well and mobile. He should be able to dress himself, attend meals and use a toilet. Some degree of disability is, however, usually present and recent evidence points to the increasing age and frailty of residents in old people's homes.

An elderly person is assessed by a social worker prior to

The elderly

Assessed by a
social worker

admission into residential Part 3 accommodation. Normally, all efforts are made to keep the person in his/her own home if possible, especially if this is what the elderly person wants. This, however, may cause considerable conflict between the general practitioner and the social worker, the doctor preferring the old person to be in a home where he is not at risk of falls or neglect.

Financial
arrangements

Once an old person enters a local authority home permanently, he has security of tenure and can stay there until he dies or is admitted into hospital. Financial arrangements vary but as the costs are high, the old person will normally be expected to contribute depending on his income, resources and capital. This may mean selling his home to raise the money for the fees. Thus, entering a home is not a decision to be taken lightly by anyone concerned. Voluntary organizations like the Elderly Invalids Fund and Distressed Gentlefolk's Association can sometimes help with the fees. In privately run homes, financial help can sometimes be obtained from the local authority or the DHSS.

Conflict of interests

Division
between
medical and
social services

Great problems can also arise as the care of frail old people is divided between the hospital services, the primary care team and social services. All may have different viewpoints, wishes and priorities. Thus the local social services department may consider an old person needs hospital care while the hospital services disagree. Lack of co-ordination and co-operation may also result in a lack of continuity of care, elderly people being discharged from hospital without the knowledge of the community services.

Co-operation
vital

The local authority may also lack resources such as places in old people's homes, thus hospital beds are used when other accommodation is more appropriate. Conversely, many old people in local residential accommodation need considerable nursing care. Co-operation between services is vital as well as a flexible approach to caring.

Compulsory removal from home

Local authorities, on the written advice of specially appointed medical practitioners, do have powers to remove people to

<table>
<tr><td>Compulsory
removal</td><td>hospital or some suitable place, but this action is rarely taken.</td></tr>
</table>

Compulsory removal

hospital or some suitable place, but this action is rarely taken. Only those living in really bad conditions and refusing to be cared for at home can be removed. The social services department has to apply for a Removal Order from the local magistrate.

Normally 7 days notice must be given to the person involved, although immediate action can be taken in emergencies. The Court Order lasts for 3 months (3 weeks for emergency Orders) but further periods of time can be granted. These powers are only taken by the local authority with great reluctance.

Financial problems

A noticeable feature of the research into poverty is how prominent the elderly are. Townsend and Wedderburn in their survey of 4000 people found that, in general, the elderly had income levels a half or more below the levels of younger people in the population. Over one third were solely dependent on state benefits. The very old were the worst off because of inflation and because they were less likely to work. Single and widowed women were also likely to be the poorest.

Apart from savings and private investment, the main sources of income are likely to be one or more of the following: (1) pensions provided through employers' superannuation schemes, (2) pensions provided through private insurance, (3) national insurance retirement pensions, (4) supplementary benefit/pension, and (5) grants from charities and benevolent funds.

The main source of income for most elderly people, however, is national insurance and supplementary pensions. Few old people have much in the way of savings and occupational pensions tend to be small in value.

Non-take-up of benefits

There is, however, mounting evidence that many old people are living on smaller incomes than the scales provided by the Supplementary Benefits Commission. A study based on 1975 estimates concluded that nearly one million people, of which over 60% were pensioners, were not receiving the supplementary benefit to which they were entitled. The main reasons why pensioners do not apply for assistance were found to be lack of knowledge, dislike of charity, a feeling that they were managing all right and a dislike of applying for it. Pensioners should be encouraged to apply for help as they can be easily put off trying by any rudeness or unhelpfulness of the first person they approach.

Need encouragement to apply

Pensions

Retirement

Shortly before retiring, the patient should receive forms from the DHSS but if not, he should apply to his local office. A retirement pension is payable to people of pensionable age (60 for women, 65 for men) provided they have paid sufficient national insurance contributions and have retired from regular full-time work. Anyone over 80 who satisfies certain residence conditions is entitled to a non-contributory pension. (Further details of this and supplementary benefit are to be found in the section on financial problems.)

Supplementary benefit

Social
security

Patients on retirement pensions may also be eligible for additional financial assistance from the Supplementary Benefits Commission if their income does not reach a minimum amount. Additions to the basic supplementary pension may be given for heating, special diets, laundry, etc. Single lump sum payments may also be given for furniture, household equipment, repairs and redecoration of accommodation, removal expenses, funeral expenses and fares to visit relatives in hospital, etc.

Other help available

Help with
health charges

Pensioners and others are entitled to help with certain NHS charges, such as free prescriptions, reduced or free charges for glasses, dentures, dental treatment, etc. Persons receiving supplementary benefit can claim refunds of their fares when attending hospital for treatment.

Help with
housing costs

Pensioners may be eligible for financial help from their local authority in the form of rate rebates, rent rebates and rent allowances. They should apply to their local authority for the appropriate forms. Pensioners on supplementary pensions are usually not entitled to these rebates as their pension covers the rates. It is often advisable for a pensioner to visit the Citizens' Advice Bureau (or welfare right officer) to investigate whether he will be better off claiming supplementary benefit or housing rebates.

Housing
repairs

Those receiving supplementary benefit may sometimes be given money towards the cost of housing repairs but usually this sum is inadequate for major repairs. The local authority

69

may lend money to owner occupiers who are unable to obtain a mortgage to cover repairs. Details are available from the appropriate local authority.

Free travel and other concessions

Some local authorities have schemes of free or reduced travel fares for elderly people. Many other authorities and commercial establishments have special concessions for old age pensioners, such as free further education courses. Details may be found from local Citizens' Advice Bureaux, the WRVS, consumer advice centres or old people's welfare associations.

Information regarding widow's benefit, death grants, attendance and invalid care allowance are listed in Chapter 9.

Additional financial help

Help from voluntary services

People may also receive financial help from voluntary sources (some of which are listed in the Appendices). As there is an enormous range of charitable trusts, some linked with individual trades or professions, the services, particular illnesses and disabilities, it may be easiest to refer the patient to the local Citizens' Advice Bureau or the local social services department. There is, however, an official central register of charities and published directories which can be found in public libraries.

Housing problems

Most elderly people live in homes of their own, rather than in any form of residential care. Approximately 89% live in ordinary accommodation, 5% in sheltered housing and only 6% live in some form of institution such as an old persons' home or hospital. A lower proportion of the elderly than all householders are owner occupiers. More are local authority or housing association tenants and a higher proportion rent private accommodation.

Adequacy and amenities

Adequate housing is of major importance to the elderly. Such features as the presence of an indoor lavatory may enable even a very frail person to continue living independently. Warmth,

The elderly

too, is particularly necessary for less active people. Familiar surroundings and nearness to shops, post office, pub and church also contribute to their ability to live alone.

A recent survey found that nearly 70% of dwellings occupied by elderly heads of households were in good condition but the standards were markedly below average among householders aged 85 or over. Many elderly people are inadequately housed, often lacking a hot water supply, an inside toilet or bathroom; 30% of bedrooms occupied by the elderly have been found to be unheated. There is evidence, too, that some people remain in residential care only because alternative adequate accommodation is lacking. Generally, the older and poorer the household, the fewer the amenities.

There are often problems because the housing occupied by the elderly person or couple is too large and too difficult to manage. Large homes bring problems of repairs, heating, decorating and cleaning. However, it is often not easy for an elderly person to change his accommodation if he is in council or private accommodation.

Sheltered housing

There are many advantages to sheltered housing. The elderly person has his own flat with a warden on hand for emergencies. sometimes there are communal eating and meeting facilities and laundering. Many have intercom and alarm bell systems. The warden's job is basically that of a good neighbour who will summon the assistance of services and relatives, if necessary. He is not expected to give any nursing or domestic help.

Although sheltered housing has been seen as having a preventive role reducing the need for Part 3 accommodation, there are problems associated with having groups of elderly people all together with no intermixing of ages. Problems also arise when tenants become older and more frail and should be in some form of residential care. These problems can be reduced if the tenants can be given extra forms of help, such as home nursing.

Details of sheltered accommodation can be obtained from the social services department.

Other types of housing

There are a number of housing associations who provide for the needs of the elderly, sometimes including sheltered housing.

Housing associations
The social services department will have details and may help in contacting these.

Hostels
Hostels are another type of provision. One variety is provided by the 300 or so Abbeyfield Societies where 8–10 elderly people live in bedsitters in one house with a housekeeper cooking meals.

Granny annexes
There have also been a number of schemes developed by local authorities and private firms where self-contained units for an elderly relative are built next to family dwellings. Alternatively, part of the family's home can be converted to a granny annexe.

Some health-related issues
Poor nutrition

Extent of problem
While the early poverty studies showed that many old people did not enjoy a diet which enabled them to remain healthy, more recent evidence suggests that there is now little overt undernutrition. However, it is sometimes necessary to assess whether an old person is getting adequate nourishment and to advise on proper food intake. Those who are apathetic, depressed, living alone and disabled are most at risk. Other risk factors include ill-fitting dentures or difficulties in shopping.

Local authority provision
A home help or meals on wheels may be invaluable. If the person is able to get out, a luncheon club may be the answer. A person may regain his or her appetite with company. Additional allowances are available from the DHSS for

Financial assistance
dietary problems, for example, diabetics or those with peptic ulcers.

Incontinence

Stress on relatives
It is estimated that two million people of all ages, many of them elderly, suffer from incontinence. Unfortunately, many people do not ask for assistance because of embarrassment. It does have social consequences as it can lay great stress on relatives and may be a determining factor as to whether a family will care for a person.

Services and financial assistance
Local authorities can supply aids, such as disposable pads, or protective bedding, and provide laundry services. The DHSS can pay a special needs allowance to cover extra laundry costs.

Hypothermia

Risk factors

Although there is no simple way of identifying those in the coldest homes, it does seem that the very elderly, poor, house- or bedbound individuals in inadequate housing are most at risk of hypothermia, especially if they are socially isolated and neglect themselves.

Many of those 'at risk' are unlikely to report that they feel cold and require warmer conditions. A survey published in 1978 found that high proportions of elderly had no means of heating their bedrooms and that a majority of halls, passages, and lavatories and many kitchens were unheated. Households with heads aged 85 or over were in many respects worse off.

What can be done

Training necessary to identify 'at risk' patients

Reports and pamphlets have recommended publicity about the extent of the problem, more financial help towards heating costs, greater attention to housing in the elderly, more insulation and a change of attitudes of fuel boards towards debt and disconnection. Certainly there is a need for training for all those in contact with the elderly, especially home helps and nursing staff, to be aware of symptoms and to be able to identify individuals most at risk. The elderly should be encouraged to live and sleep in one room, if necessary, with adequate clothing such as bedsocks and headwear.

The psychological and social needs of the dying

Although about one half of terminally ill people appear to appreciate the seriousness of their illness, this awareness is usually achieved informally and indirectly. One survey found that only 15% of terminally ill cancer patients were told of their prognosis by the doctors concerned. By contrast, 90% of the close relatives were told by a member of the medical profession.

Whether to tell

One study found that dying patients welcomed talking about the possibilities of death to a sympathetic listener and were glad to discuss their fears. The patient may have no one to confide in, being unable to talk openly to their spouse. It is always a difficult decision about whether to tell the patient the truth about his prognosis. It is important to listen carefully to the patient's wishes and questions on this matter as well as those of the relatives. A person who knows can hopefully come to terms with his own death, make certain adjustments and prepare himself for the inevitable.

In general, learning that one has a fatal illness is followed by a period of disquiet, similar to a grief reaction, although this response may be concealed. At first, the patient may be shocked, numbed and deny the possibility. He may search for alternative medical help or seek a second opinion. A deep sense of isolation is also common. Anger often follows with feelings of rage, envy and resentment. Later, the patient may start to bargain, trying to postpone his death by promising to be good either secretly to God or to others. As the patient gradually realizes his fate, he is likely to become depressed and withdrawn. Finally, most patients (but not all) achieve some sort of peace before the end, accepting the inevitable. During this period, the family may need more help than the patient.

Stages of adjustment

The patient needs to undergo a major psychological adjustment to accept his own death which takes time but is helped by the empathy and caring of others. The psychological needs of a dying patient should be as central a concern as the physical, the patient being given time to talk about his fears and griefs. Anxiety is also very common but its relief as well as the relief of depression can reduce the amount of physical pain felt by patients. This in turn can reduce the dosages of pain-relieving drugs which are necessary.

Psychological needs

Support for the family

The doctor has to consider the welfare of the survivors before they become bereaved. The distress, depression and anxiety may be as great or greater for them as the sufferer himself. The community nursing services will provide nursing care for the patient dying at home and may give much general support and encouragement to the family. The local authority social worker can also help by practical assistance such as providing aids, laundry services and by offering counselling help. Many people turn towards the clergy who can help the patient and the family both before the death and afterwards. Voluntary organizations can also assist, many helping specific illnesses (see the appendices).

Other services

Loss of a spouse in old age can be a severe blow to the survivor and most old people never really get over it. They may become withdrawn, depressed, apathetic and socially isolated. They may neglect themselves, lose weight and be at risk of becoming ill and dying themselves. Often they cope better if they prepare themselves for their bereavement before the actual death occurs.

Bereavement among the elderly

Summary of the services and help available

This list includes the range of help which may be available, although in practice the extent of provision varies considerably depending on the geographical area.

Agency	*Type of help*
Local authority social services department. These services are normally arranged by a social worker or another member of the department such as the home help organizer	Social work help including advice, assistance, information and emotional support
	Home helps
	Meals-on-wheels/luncheon clubs
	Recreational facilities, day centres and social clubs
	Help with transport and bus passes
	Aids and adaptations to the home (including a telephone under certain circumstances)
	Laundry services
	Holidays
	Sheltered housing, lodgings and boarding-out schemes
	Short- and long-term residential care
	Financial assistance (through applying to charities)
Local education authority	Day and evening classes for recreational and educational activities (including courses on retirement)
Local offices of the Department of Health and Social Security	Financial help including the following benefits: retirement pensions, widows pensions, supplementary benefit, disability benefits

Summary of services and help available (continued)

Voluntary agencies	Social and leisure activities including outings
	Transport
	Aids and adaptations
	Holidays
	Financial help
	Specialized housing and residential homes (including the work of housing associations)
	Sheltered work centres
	Volunteers to visit and help with domestic chores and shopping

The physically disabled

The physically disabled

The term 'physically disabled' encompasses people of all ages who are disabled before or through birth, through illness, injury, blindness or deafness. As many of the physically disabled are also elderly, there will be considerable overlap between this chapter and that on the elderly and many of the associations and services apply to both.

The most detailed source of information on the population of people with disabilities in Britain was conducted in 1968/1969. Although there have been many efforts to define the concept of disability, for the purposes of this survey, *impairment* was defined as lacking part or all of a limb, or having a defective limb, organ or mechanism of the body, *disablement* was the loss or reduction of functional ability, and *handicap* was the disadvantage or restriction of activity caused by disability. This survey estimated that there were 3 million impaired people aged 16 or over in private households in Great Britain including some 1.1 million severely or appreciably handicapped people. Estimates suggested that this figure has increased since 1968 and that the survey, for a variety of reasons, underestimated the incidence of disability. Other estimates suggest as many as 9.9 million people are impaired included 3 million handicapped.

The proportion of people who will become disabled in the course of their lives is very high indeed. By their early seventies, over a fifth of men and a quarter of women are appreciably or severely disabled. High numbers of people are

Definition of terms

Estimates of numbers disabled

Higher numbers affected by disability

affected directly or indirectly by disability, through having a child, a spouse, parent or other relative with a disability.

With increases in the elderly population, the emphasis on community care and recent medical advances, the numbers of disabled people living in the community are constantly rising. This increases the responsibility of the primary care team and the local authority towards the disabled.

Increased responsibility for the GP

Although various changes in society have meant that there is a smaller number of people available to care for the disabled, there has been a marked improvement in the situation of disabled people in the United Kingdom over the last decade. Twenty years ago, few disabled people were seen in public. Now, there are reserved parking spaces for cars, ramped entrances to buildings, adapted toilets. Disabled people are more readily accepted as part of the community and enter more into its social relations. They are now considered to have the same rights as the non-disabled and more have come forward to express their views and describe their problems. This explains the sudden spurt in consumer and self-help groups.

Better public acceptance

Social and psychological problems

People with disabilities have a variety of personal and social problems. They are more likely than non-disabled to be living on or below the poverty line, to experience housing problems, lack basic amenities, have dietary deficiencies and experience social deprivation. They are less likely to go out socially, are less mobile and have fewer interests and activities.

There are a variety of services to cater for the needs of the disabled – government departments, local authorities and voluntary agencies. There are large numbers of different voluntary organizations, some catering for very specific disabilities, others more general. Many have local branches or representatives to provide advice, assistance and support.

Problems adjusting to disability

After a person becomes disabled, his personality must alter to come into line with his changed status or role in life and his altered body image. He also has to adjust to being treated differently by others.

Writers have suggested that disabled people go through a

Adjustment to disability

process similar to grieving or mourning. First, there is shock, then denial, the person refusing to accept that recovery will not take place, followed by anger and then depression. However, individuals do vary, some become depressed many years after disability. The individual's reaction will depend very much on his particular social situation, on the reaction of his family or friends, and on the attitudes of the professionals involved, his doctor, the hospital staff, etc. It will also depend on other social factors, whether he can still continue in employment and whether he can carry on with the same recreational activities. The doctor's role may be crucial in supporting him through this period.

Relationships within the family

Strains on the family

The family's needs

The precise impact of disablement on family life depends on the position of the disabled person within the family. However, one disabled member will have an effect on the relationships and opportunities of the family as a whole. Thus, a disabled child may place great strains on his parent's marriage and may lead to behaviour problems in the other siblings. Adjustment to sudden traumatic disability may be harder for the other members of the family than the disabled person. Allowances and sympathy may be extended to the disabled person whereas others are simply expected to cope. The family's needs should be considered by the professionals involved.

Marital adjustment

Marital problems

A disabled man or women has to reshape his or her marital role to take account of the disability but spouses also have to adjust their role correspondingly. A husband of a disabled wife may find that a great deal of time is spent on domestic duties which may affect his work and his occupational satisfaction. This may lead to lost job opportunities and fewer chances of promotion. A husband with a disabled wife may also find he misses not being able to go out with her so often. These factors may account for the higher rate of marital breakdown when the wife is disabled than when the husband is. There is usually financial hardship when the husband is disabled but the wife's new role may not need so much psychological adjustment on her part. Her roles in life are more domestic and she is used to caring for dependants and may thus be more able to cope with the restrictions imposed by her husband's disability.

Sexual problems

Sexual needs

The sexual needs of the disabled are often not recognized. The general public sometimes refuse to accept that the severely handicapped have sexual feelings and consider that relationships between members of the opposite sex should be discouraged or denied.

Self-image disturbed

For someone disabled after marriage, the impact on the sexual relationship may be far more severe than the actual degree of functional loss. The self-image of the disabled person is likely to be severely affected, they may consider themselves sexually unattractive and refuse to believe that their spouse still cares for them sexually, causing them to reject their spouse's advances. Disabled women are more likely to be affected as physical attractiveness is usually more important to their self-image. Those suddenly disabled in accidents are more likely to have sexual difficulties. In a slowly progressing disease, the couple have time to adjust and change their outlook gradually.

The single disabled person also has problems. He or she may have few opportunities to meet the opposite sex and may have problems in forming a relationship with another person, doubting his or her sexual attractiveness.

Physical difficulties

Apart from these problems, there may also be physical difficulties too. The person may be rendered impotent or partially impotent or there may be difficulties in performance due to the impairment.

The role of the doctor

The doctor is in an important position to help and offer advice or refer the patient on to another agency if necessary. He must not overlook these problems in his disabled patients and offer sympathy and support as well as practical advice on how best to overcome them. Voluntary agencies for the disabled can offer help for these problems and a special group has been set up to give general help and advice as well as promoting understanding in this area (address in the Appendices).

Problems of having a handicapped child (including the mentally handicapped)

Reliable information on the national prevalence of children who are handicapped or impaired is not available. Estimates vary widely but surveys and cohorts suggest that more than 500 000 children have an impairment of some sort.

The multiple handicaps of more severely disabled children place considerable restrictions on their families far more than those of non-disabled children and for considerably longer. In practice, most of the work falls on the mother but the quality of life of the whole family is usually affected.

The first shock of learning

Many parents retrospectively comment on the unsatisfactory way that medical and social work staff avoided confronting them with the truth. They consider it important to be given clear factual information as soon as possible, although some account should be taken of each parent's individual strengths. The truth can sometimes bring relief, the parents sensing something is wrong.

The initial shock period

It may be helpful for the parents to have a number of sessions with someone available to give repeated explanations and information. If possible, one person such as a health visitor or social worker, should provide regular and sustained contact with the family to help them over the initial distressing period.

Reaction of parent

Parents will feel a mixture of feelings at first, shock, anger, guilt, grief and embarrassment. They need empathy and understanding and should be given the opportunity to express their bitterness and resentment. Their personal assets and strengths need to be built up and encouraged.

After the initial shock, parents may still be very rejecting or they may become too overprotecting. Many mothers become totally involved in their handicapped child, keeping him in babyish dependence and excluding the involvement of others.

Worries about the future

After the early shock of learning about the child's disability, there will be a number of worries about the child's health, survival and future. As the child matures, there will be worries over sexual needs and activities and there is often a difficult period when a change is made from school to the training centre. The parents will worry about the child's prospects for work or marriage. They will be concerned about what happens when they become too old to cope or die. In addition, the parents and siblings may also feel the stigma of having a handicapped child in the family and find difficulties in making friends.

Having a physically or mentally handicapped child can also

be sheer physical hard work. The child may need to be lifted,
The work carried, bathed, dressed and fed and as he gets older and
involved heavier these tasks become harder. The parents' mental and
emotional energies may be drained by broken nights or
behaviour problems. As the child gets older, his disabilities
become more apparent as the gap between him and his non-
disabled peers widens.

As the handicapped child will need a considerable amount of
Effect on care, less time is available for the siblings or the spouse. It is
family usually leisure and recreational activities that suffer most,
family outings may be impossible, especially if there is no easy
means of transport. In addition, neighbours and friends may be
unwilling to babysit to give parents a night out.

Given these anxieties and the physical day-to-day care, it is
High levels of not surprising that mothers of severely disabled children have
stress and repeatedly been found to suffer from high levels of stress and
marital stress-related illness. There is also a high rate of marital break-
breakdown down and family problems, other family members resenting the
lack of time given to them and the restrictions imposed on
going out and leisure time.

The family doctor is a key position to support and encourage
The role of the the family. It is important that he allows the family to give vent
doctor and to their feelings which are often ambivalent. However, help
voluntary from voluntary agencies such as MENCAP and self-help groups
agencies can be particularly important, parents receiving and giving
sympathy to families in a similar position. Details of
organizations are given in the Appendices or are available from
the social services department.

Problems of rehabilitation and managing at home

Most general hospitals have rehabilitation departments where
disabled people after an accident or illness can obtain artificial
limbs, eyes, hearing aids, surgical supports, invalid chairs,
Rehabilitation vehicles and other appliances. In addition, there are also
department special demonstration centres. After the patient is discharged
from hospital, the local authority social workers should be able
to assist the patient to obtain the services, enabling him to
manage at home.

The role of the local authority

The Chronically Sick and Disabled Persons Act 1970 obliges
local authorities to ascertain the number of disabled people

living in their area and to provide them with social services, many of which enable them to continue living at home or with their families.

The services they should provide are similar to those listed

Services provided

for the elderly. They include:

(1) Practical assistance in the home including the home help service.

(2) Meals (meals-on-wheels or luncheon clubs).

(3) Wireless, television or library facilities.

(4) Recreational facilities including outings, day centres, social clubs, sheltered employment and holidays. Transport should also be available.

(5) Adaptation to the home including telephones. Telephones should be available to isolated housebound individuals who may need urgent medical help. The rental may also be partly paid.

Charges

A charge may be made for any of the above services but some local authorities provide these services free.

Variation in the extent of provision

Local authorities, however, vary enormously in the services they provide and how they interpret the Act. Thus, what a disabled person receives will depend very much on the locality in which he lives. In practice, most services are given to the elderly and few are given to the disabled person under 65 who still has to depend on his family for his care. Although, in theory, the local authority should offer a wide range of services for the disabled, only a minority receive any benefit.

Registration

Although the local authority is required to keep a register of all physically disabled people in its area, registration is no longer compulsory as it is not a prerequisite for assistance. Medical advice may be required by the local authority to determine the classification of the disability for registration purposes.

Aids to mobility

Aids to mobility

Mobility is vital to enable a disabled person to remain in and integrate with the community. Responsibility for supplying the disabled with limbs, wheelchairs, cars, etc., rests with the regional artificial limb and appliance centres under the DHSS. A doctor or social worker must apply on the patient's behalf. Nominations for a car have to be made by a hospital consultant. Cars normally are only available to those who cannot walk and need mobility to secure or keep employment, look after a family or pursue a study or training course. Other aids to mobility are generally arranged through the nursing services or the physiotherapist.

Aids in the home

Adaptation to the home

The local authority has the responsibility to provide aids or adapt the housing so that the disabled person can manage at home. Again, local authorities vary widely, some carrying out major adaptations such as installing a lift or constructing a downstairs lavatory. However, the home adaptations that are carried out are nearly always minor, such as fixing hand rails to the bath or the stairs. House renovation grants (improvement or intermediate grants) may also be made available to disabled people for adapting their homes. Local authority tenants should go to the housing or social services department for help. If the housing department carries out the adaptation the rent may be increased.

Personal hygiene and domestic aids

A wide range of aids are also available for activities such as toileting, washing, shaving, dressing, feeding and other domestic tasks. The local authority and voluntary organizations can provide these. An exhibition of the variety of aids available can be seen at the Disabled Living Foundation's headquarters (see Appendix 5). However, a number of books describe and illustrate the range of aids available.

Other domiciliary services

The role of social workers, occupational and speech therapists

The disabled person can be seen at home by an occupational therapist who can help the patient cope with the tasks of day-to-day living. If the patient has problems with his speech, he can receive help from a speech therapist. Social workers will visit disabled people in their own homes to give advice and information about local services and to assess the need of a particular service. On a long-term basis, social workers can provide support and help to the disabled person and his family.

Housing problems

The majority of disabled people live in private households rather than residential care. However, disability creates special needs and many disabled people are unsuitably housed. A government survey estimated that a quarter of impaired people need substantial improvement to their accommodation or rehousing. Only 5% of the disabled live in purpose built accommodation for the elderly or disabled and nearly all of these are elderly persons.

Specialized accommodation for the less severely disabled

Specially built accommo-
dation sheltered housing

Although local authorities have been charged with the responsibility of taking into account the needs of the disabled in future housing plans, specialized housing is only increasing slowly and demand still very much exceeds supply. However, many local authorities do have specially adapted council housing for those who do not need supervision, as well as sheltered accommodation with a resident warden for those who might need occasional assistance. In addition, some local authorities have initiated schemes for placing the disabled in lodgings with a landlady or family for those who cannot live independently. Details of these schemes are available from the local authority social services department or from the housing department.

Boarding out

Housing associations and voluntary agencies

Some housing associations also specialize in accommodation for the disabled while others cater for the able-bodied and disabled on an integrated basis. Many voluntary organizations have their own range of accommodation catering for different degrees of disability. A social worker from the local authority should be able to assist in applying for the local authority provision and in giving details of relevant housing associations and voluntary organizations.

Residential services

The most severely disabled who cannot live with their own family will need permanent residential care. The local authority has the responsibility to provide for them if they are not ill. Sick people needing hospital treatment are the responsibility of the National Health Service. In practice, for the severely disabled there is a fine dividing line between whether he needs a hospital or a residential placement, leading to arguments over who is responsible for care. This has a direct effect on the cost to the patient or family, the NHS provision being free while that provided by the local authority is usually not. Local authorities usually fix standard charges related to actual costs and the resident pays according to his or her means. Those with a low income can claim supplementary benefit, however.

Charges

The provision of residential accommodation varies throughout the country but generally social services departments are making less use of the accommodation provided in the vast old institutions inherited from the old public assistance authorities. Increasingly, accommodation is being provided in small homes and hostels built especially for the purpose or produced by the conversion of existing large houses.

Type of accommo-
dation
available

Educational problems

Parents of a handicapped child face the dilemma about whether their child will do better in a special school adapted to their particular needs or integrated in a normal school. At this particular time, the emphasis of educational authorities is to include as many physically handicapped children into ordinary schools as possible. This has the advantage of teaching the child how to manage and cope with 'normal society' and he can make friends with non-handicapped children. However, this can be more stressful for the disabled child who feels different and who may not be accepted readily. Evidence suggests that those with severe handicaps do better in special schools where the teaching and environment is geared to their particular needs. A boarding school may be necessary for the severely handicapped, for those needing a specialist school that serves a large area or if home conditions are poor.

Integrate or
segregate

The education of all school age children is the responsibility of the local education authority who will be involved in the choice of school for any handicapped child. The local education office will have details of facilities in the area or of residential provision. The child's need for special education may be assessed by educational psychologists, medical officers, social workers and teaching staff. Although most boarding schools are maintained by voluntary organizations, the local education authority will pay the tuition fees and boarding school fees if they assess that pupils should be sent to these schools. The educational welfare officer can be contacted for help with the practical details such as transport or for any other matter concerning the child's welfare.

Responsibility
of the local
education
authority

Education
welfare officer

86

The physically disabled

Problems of employment

The disabled wish to spend their time constructively as much as the non-disabled and gather the same satisfactions from being gainfully employed. The majority of disabled people of working age become disabled due to disease or injury after entering the labour force and many of these can still keep in the same employment, after making some adjustments. However, many disabled have severe difficulties both in obtaining employment and when at work. Fewer are employed than the non-disabled; in 1981, 16% of the registered disabled were unemployed in comparison with 8% of the total workforce. This percentage is likely to be an underestimate as many disabled do not register as unemployed, knowing that there is little chance of work. When at work, the disabled earn less than the non-disabled, are generally in less responsible positions and have poorer conditions of work.

The Employment Service agency and the Training Service agency are the two government bodies which play an important role in finding suitable employment for the disabled.

The DRO and the Disabled Persons Employment Register

The DRO

Disabled persons who wish to work may either apply for work on the open market or register as disabled. There are specialist officers in the employment offices, called Disablement Resettlement Officers (DRO) who can offer advice and assistance to the disabled.

Disabled Persons Employment Register

The Disabled Persons Employment Register is open to all people whose disabilities handicap them in obtaining employment. There are two categories, those capable of working in general employment and those more severely handicapped who can only work in sheltered workshops.

Quota scheme

Those capable of general employment may be able to obtain employment through the quota scheme. Under the scheme, any employer of more than 20 persons is required to take up to 3% of his staff from disabled persons on the register. Until the quota is filled, an employer may not fill any vacancies with an able-bodied person. Unfortunately, in practice, the system is usually not enforced, although there are provisions for prosecutions and penalties.

The DRO will have details of jobs through this scheme. In addition, certain occupations such as passenger lift operators and car park attendants are reserved for the registered disabled.

87

Problems in social care

Sheltered
employment
and Remploy

Those persons who are severely disabled or near retirement age and cannot find employment can be trained for work in a sheltered workshop. The government runs its own schemes in a number of Remploy factories and local authorities and voluntary organizations also provide workshops. Earnings are low, however, and there is a shortage of available places. In addition, the severely handicapped are sometimes not considered acceptable even though they may wish to work.

Stigma of
being disabled

Only half of those eligible to register do so. This is because many people consider that registration does little to help in obtaining employment and can even be a hindrance because of the stigma attached to being disabled. Others try the open market to secure employment, many concealing their disability. Disabled persons are able to remove their names from the register if they wish.

Assessment for working capacity

Medical
assessment

Employment services often require a medical assessment so that they have some idea of the individual's capacity for working. When a more detailed assessment is desirable, the person can be admitted to an industrial rehabilitation unit, recommended by the DRO, doctor or hospital. Here, the person's potential is assessed and he is given advice and help.

Eligibility for
training
courses

Disabled persons are also eligible to apply for a course at a vocational training centre or a residential centre. However, places are limited.

Problems with mobility, transport and social activities

The disabled go out less frequently than the non-disabled; most outdoor trips are restricted to essential shopping or visiting friends or relatives. Like the elderly, the disabled are often isolated and lonely. Few make use of the recreational services available to them through the local authority. There are, however, many specialist clubs for the disabled and many sport centres provide activities for the disabled. Voluntary organiz-

Voluntary
provision

ations can be helpful and the British Sports Association for the Disabled can give individual advice from their local representatives. In addition, there are a number of clubs supplying contacts, talking books, newspapers or tapes, etc. which may be useful to the housebound.

Voluntary organizations, as well as the local authorities, also

Specialist
holidays

arrange a number of holidays for the disabled. There are a number of specialist holiday centres (e.g. riding holidays for the disabled) and the Family Fund can give financial help for holidays for families with handicapped children. A comprehensive guide to these holidays is published annually by RADAR (address in Appendix 5).

Travel
arrangements

Social services departments generally provide transport to clubs, centres and workshops for disabled people who are unable to use public transport. For those who can travel independently there are various schemes administered by social services departments to enable the disabled to travel either free or at a reduced rate on public transport, and to enable cars with disabled drivers or passengers to park more easily by displaying special orange car badges.

Financial problems

Extra expense
entailed

Disablement often entails financial disadvantage. The proportion of people with disabilities aged 15 or over living in or close to poverty is three times that for the non-disabled. If the disabled person is the breadwinner, the disablement may result in loss of employment or reduction in earning capacity. If the disabled person is the spouse or child, the disablement may cause loss of a second income, and additional domestic help may be necessary. In addition, disablement usually involves extra expenses, for heating, transport, visits to hospitals, domestic or maintenance chores, etc. Thus, a below average income for a family with a disabled member implies a great more hardship than the same income going to an able-bodied household.

Most are
reliant on
state benefits

The majority of disabled people do not work and are reliant on state benefits for at least part of their income. The principal sources of income are retirement pensions, supplementary benefit, invalidity pensions, industrial injury and war pensions.

In addition to the benefits payable to the non-disabled, the disabled are eligible for a number of other allowances. Those with disabled children are eligible for mobility and attendance allowances or help from the Family Fund.

National insurance invalidity benefit

Benefits
available

This is payable to those with a contribution record at the full rate. The rate is a little higher than the standard supplementary benefit level. Few married women are eligible as the majority do not pay full rate national insurance contributions.

Non-contributory invalidity pension

This was introduced in 1975. It is payable to those below retirement age who are unable to work due to disability and who do not have a national insurance contribution record. Married women are also excluded unless they can show that they are unable to work and unable to perform normal household duties. This pension is of value to only a small proportion of the disabled who are not eligible to claim supplementary benefit, such as those with an income from savings or a private pension. Those claiming supplementary benefit will have the invalidity pension deducted from the benefit.

Married women excluded

Attendance allowance

This is available to those so severely disabled as to need continuous attention by day or by night or both. It is also payable for a child of 2 or older who needs substantially more care or supervision than an able-bodied child of the same age or sex. It is tax free, not dependent on a contribution record and disregarded in calculating entitlement to other benefit. It is payable at two rates according to whether help is necessary both day and night or only one of these periods.

Allowances for the severely disabled

Mobility allowance

This is payable to disabled adults under retirement age or children over 5 who are unable or virtually unable to walk. It is a non-contributory, non-means tested benefit but is taxable.

Invalid care allowance

This allowance is payable to those, *other than married women*, who give up work to care for a disabled person in receipt of an attendance allowance. As with the non-contributory invalidity pension, individuals are credited with national insurance contributions while in receipt of these benefits, thus safeguarding future entitlements.

Allowance for 'carers'

90

The physically disabled

The Family Fund

This was set up in 1973 to complement existing provision from statutory and voluntary services for families with disabled children. To be eligible, a child has to be very severely disabled, aged under 16 and living at home. By the end of 1980, the fund had distributed £18.8 million to families for items like washing machines and driers, transport, clothing, bedding, and holidays. Families ask the Fund for things they need to relieve stress and the Fund responds to their requests using its own discretion rather than strict rules of eligibility. This means that some families have received considerably less help than others. Details of help are available from the local authority social services department.

Extra help for those with handicapped children

Help from voluntary organizations

A number of charities and voluntary agencies can assist disabled people in buying items such as washing machines etc. or in paying off accumulated debts. The social worker in the social services department should be able to help in writing to these agencies or the Citizens' Advice Bureau in giving details of charities.

Services for the blind and partially sighted

The blind have special needs and therefore have additional services available to them as well as those for the physically disabled.

The local social services departments are responsible for compiling a register of all blind and partially sighted people. There are two distinct categories of registration – the blind and the partially sighted. The definition of blindness is 'that a person should be so blind as to be unable to perform any work for which eyesight is essential'. Registration is voluntary but is a prerequisite for certain financial benefits including an addition to the supplementary benefit rate. A certificate of registration is completed by a consultant or ophthalmologist and forwarded to the local social services department.

Registration of the blind

Extra financial benefit

There is no statutory definition of partial sight. A person who is not entitled to be registered as blind but who is substantially and permanently handicapped by defective vision is within the scope of the welfare services that local authorities are

Partial sight

91

empowered to provide for blind persons. This provision does not, however, extend to the financial benefits which are available for registered blind people.

Social work with the blind

The role of the
social worker

The local authority social worker is responsible for co-ordinating the statutory and voluntary services for the blind. Most local authorities employ staff who specialize in this work. The social worker's task is to visit the blind or partially sighted person to give advice and information about registration and the local services available, and support the individual and his family in coping with the effects of blindness. If specially qualified, the social worker, where appropriate, may teach mobility, reading and writing by tactile methods, and the use of aids and equipment which may help the visually handicapped to communicate with others and control their enviroment.

Other facilities

Equipment
and aids

Special designed equipment and aids are available from social services departments. The Royal National Institute for the Blind (RNIB) publishes a catalogue of equipment and items may be obtained direct from them. The blind also receive special concessions for radio and television and reduced television licence fees. They can receive books and periodicals in braille and large print books are available from many libraries.

Guide dogs

In addition, blind people can attend courses to receive the necessary training for a guide dog. A medical report is needed when an application is made.

Employment

There are some 30 DROs who specialize in finding employment for blind people. Some of the blind are employed on the open market as typists, telephonists or in executive and administrative work. Others find sheltered employment which may be in specialist workshops for the blind. The specialist DROs collaborate with RNIB to find placements.

Holidays

Some social services departments provide holiday accommodation for blind and partially sighted people. Voluntary organizations for the blind such as the RNIB also have holiday hotels. The local social services department may be able to help with the cost of a holiday for a blind person.

Concessions are available on most forms of public transport.

The physically disabled

Travel

These are sometimes limited to specific purposes and may cover a blind person's guide as well as the blind person himself. The local social services department is responsible for issuing the necessary certification for these concessions.

It is the statutory responsibility of local authorities to provide residential care for the blind if necessary. Voluntary organizations also provide care which is of a more specialized nature. Details of voluntary homes can be obtained from the RNIB.

Voluntary organizations

There are a number of organizations for the blind. The Royal National Institute for the Blind is the most useful starting point for contacting the voluntary section as it gives advice as well as a wide range of services.

Services for the deaf and hard of hearing

In general, there is a lack of awareness of the problems of the deaf and hard of hearing and this is reflected in the comparative lack of special services for this group. They are eligible, however, for the range of local authority social services available for the disabled.

Few additional services available

Additional services for the deaf include the provision of aids such as flashing door bells. Some social services departments also employ social workers with special qualifications in working with the deaf. Their task is to support the handicapped person and his family and to give advice and information about local and national services. Their training equips them with techniques for communicating with the deaf without speech. The voluntary agencies which cater for the deaf are included in the appendices.

Summary of the services and help available

In addition to the services listed below, the disabled may receive help from nurses, physiotherapists, occupational therapists and speech therapists. The following agencies and organizations may provide *some* or all of the listed types of help depending on the geographical area and the patient's disabilities.

93

Agency	Type of help
Local authority social services department. These services can be arranged by a social worker or sometimes another member of the social services department.	Social work help including advice, assistance, information and emotional support
	Home helps
	Meals-on-wheels/luncheon clubs
	Recreational facilities, day centres and social clubs
	Help with transport, bus passes, car badges, etc.
	Aids and adaptations to the home (including a telephone under certain circumstances)
	Laundry services
	Holidays
	Sheltered employment and workshops
	Sheltered housing, specialized lodgings and boarding-out schemes
	Residential care (short- and long-term)
	Financial assistance (through an application to the Family Fund or to clients)
	Specialist help for the blind and the deaf
Local authority housing department	Adaptations to the home
	Specialized housing
Local education authority	Specialized schooling (including educational assessments)
	Help of the educational welfare officer for all the educational problems of the handicapped
	Day and evening classes on a range of subjects

Summary of services and help available   (continued)

Hospital rehabilitation department	All rehabilitation services including limbs, aids and modes of transport
Department of Employment (employment offices)	The services of the disablement resettlement officer including registration, sheltered workshops and training courses
	Details of job vacancies
Local offices of Department of Health and Social Security	Financial help including the following benefits: national insurance invalidity benefit non-contributory invalidity benefit attendance allowance invalid care allowance mobility allowance supplementary benefit (higher rate for the blind)
Voluntary agencies	Emotional support to patient and family
	Help with sexual problems
	Social and leisure activities (including those at home)
	Babysitting services
	Transport
	Guide dogs for the blind
	Aids and adaptations
	Holidays
	Schools including boarding schools
	Sheltered workshops
	Financial help
	Specialized housing and residential homes (including the work of housing associations)

7 Mental illness and handicap

Mental illness and handicap

Various studies have suggested that a high proportion of patients visit their family doctors for a condition diagnosed as entirely or largely psychiatric in nature. The most comprehensive research is that carried out by Shepherd and his colleagues in 46 practices in the London area. Table 1 gives the consulting rates for different psychiatric illnesses or for psychiatric-associated conditions. After respiratory diseases, psychiatric illness was found to be the commonest reason for consulting the general practitioner. Minor mental disorders such as depression and anxiety were very frequent while severe mental disorder was seen comparatively rarely.

Extent of the problem

At all ages women are more likely to suffer from most forms of mental disorder than are men (excepting schizophrenia). For both sexes the incidence of mental disorder is highest among the divorced, separated and widowed, marriage usually offering some protection against the appearance of mental disorder. However, young married women are a particularly high-risk group, especially in their late twenties and early thirties.

Demographic characteristics

Psychiatric illnesses are likely to take up a considerable amount of the doctor's time especially as the vast majority are dealt with by the general practitioner alone, only one in 20 being referred to mental health facilities. In addition, patients with neurotic and emotional disorders make greater demands on medical care, they attend more frequently and exhibit more categories of illness per head than the remainder of patients consulting their doctors.

Time-consuming for the doctor

High attenders

97

Table 1 Patient consulting rates per 1000 at risk for psychiatric morbidity by sex and diagnostic group

Diagnostic group	Male	Female	Both sexes
Psychoses	2.7	8.6	5.9
Mental subnormality	1.6	2.9	2.3
Dementia	1.2	1.6	1.4
Neuroses	55.7	116.6	88.5
Personality disorder	7.2	4.0	5.5
Formal psychiatric illness	67.2	131.9	102.1
Psychiatric associated conditions	38.6	57.2	48.6
Total psychiatric morbidity	97.9	175.0	139.4

Source: Shepherd, M., Cooper, B., Brown, A.C. and Kalton, G.W. (1966). *Psychiatric Illness In General Practice.* (London: Oxford University Press)

The majority of the psychiatric disorders encountered in general practice are the affective disorders, including depression, anxiety or, more commonly, a mixture of them both. However, many of these illnesses are not detected by the doctor, either because the patient does not divulge his symptoms or because the doctor interprets them as part of a physical illness. This can lead to much frustration on both sides, especially if physical examinations and investigations are carried out to no avail because the underlying cause is predominantly psychological.

The importance of detection

Prognosis

Although these psychiatric illnesses take up much of the doctor's time, the bulk of them are short-lived. Longitudinal studies suggest that many are short-term reactions to a particular situation, such as a bereavement or the loss of a job. In these patients, there are often reoccurences of ill health when other problems arise. There are, however, a number of patients with more chronic disorders who will be ill for several years. As few of these patients are referred on to other facilities, they can

Prognosis

make considerable demands on the general practitioner and his time.

Social factors and psychiatric morbidity

The role of
social factors

Research studies indicate that social factors play an important part in the causation, development and severity of a patient's psychiatric illness. These social factors include stressful situations called 'life events', such as the birth of a child, as well as practical problems or interpersonal relationship difficulties. In Shepherd's study, the general practitioners were asked to record the social factors which they regarded as relevant in either the onset, course or severity of the patient's illness. In general, the doctors regarded social factors as important in the aetiology of psychiatric illness and specified no factors for only a minority of cases. They tended to report concurrent factors such as marital disharmony, housing problems and work difficulties rather than report difficulties such as childhood experiences. There was also a surprising conformity of opinion amongst the survey doctors as to which factors were more common and more important.

Social factors
and prognosis

The patient's social circumstances also affect the prognosis of psychiatric illnesses. For example, those with chronic social difficulties are less likely to recover quickly from a neurotic illness. Two recent studies have indicated that social dysfunction was the strongest single predictor of the outcome of neurotic disorder. In addition, some investigations consider that certain family dynamics not only have an important influence on the genesis and cause of schizophrenia but also determine whether a patient will relapse again once sent home.

Social
supports

While some social difficulties increase the likelihood of someone becoming ill, supportive relationships, especially with the spouse, may protect the individual either from developing a psychiatric illness or from becoming chronically ill.

Types of illness seen in general practice

The psychoses

The psychoses

These include the organic psychoses, schizophrenia, related paranoid states and manic depression. Since the widespread use of long-acting phenothiazines, lithium and other drugs,

99

patients with these illnesses are able to spend long periods in the community, the majority living with relatives. Thus, although these disorders are encountered infrequently in family practice, they do present a difficult management problem to the general practitioner and community services. The burden shouldered by relatives can be heavy and one of the major roles of the family physician in the management of such patients involves giving advice and support to the relatives. Later in this chapter, an outline will be given of some of the services available to the patient and relatives.

Emphasis is on living in the community

Non-psychotic disorders

The non-psychotic disorders constitute the bulk of the psychiatric morbidity which presents to the family physician. The majority of these illnesses are minor affective disorders in which there is often an inextricable intermingling of depression and anxiety. Anxiety can also occur on its own but this is less common. A small proportion of patients may suffer from a phobic state, anxiety amounting often to panic. These attacks can occur in the presence of specific objects, such as spiders or in certain situations, such as open spaces or heights. Obsessive, compulsive and hysterical reactions are relatively uncommon.

Depression and anxiety

Neurotic disorders are common in all age groups but may be easily overlooked in the elderly when other physical illnesses or disabilities are also present. In this age group, minor affective disorders are usually seen in the setting of serious personal and social vicissitudes such as bereavement, family breakup, social isolation or as a result of the social and physical restrictions imposed by physical illness. Difficulties in concentrating, hypochondria, disturbed sleep, apathy and loss of appetite may all be signs of depression and the patient may be a suicide risk.

Lack of recognition in the elderly

Suicide

It has been estimated that out of a hypothetical average population of 2500, there will be three suicide attempts in any 1 year and one of these will be successful every 3 years. Official statistics and studies indicate those individuals in the general population who are most at risk (Table 2). Although the suicide rate has been relatively stable in the United Kingdom, the

Suicide rates

United States and other countries over the past decade, there has been a dramatic increase in suicide attempts. Suicide attempts are most commonly made by young, divorced or single females who usually have interpersonal difficulties. By contrast, it is the depressive person over 40 years of age who is most at risk for a successful suicide attempt.

Table 2

Psychiatric illness	Depression
	Alcoholism
	Other addictions
	Early dementia
	Organic brain syndrome
Life stress	Bereavement
	Separation
	Moving house
	Loss of job
	Incapacitating physical illness
Personal aspects	Age over 40
	Male<female
	Immigrant
	Widowed, divorced, separated
	Unemployed
	Recently retired
	Socially isolated
Previous history	Family history of depression, alcoholism
	Previous history of depression, alcoholism
	Previous suicide attempt
Symptoms	Suicidal thoughts
	Ideas of guilt and unworthiness
	Lethargy and social adjustment
	Hopelessness
	Agitation and restlessness

Source: Clare, A.W. and Shepherd, M. (1978). Psychiatry and family medicine. In Fry, J., Gambrill, E. and Smith, R. (eds.). Scientific Foundations of Family Medicine. (London: Heinemann Medical Books)

The role of the GP

The general practitioner's role is clearly important since the majority of suicidal attempts are made by people taking psychotropic drugs or barbiturates often prescribed by their doctor. One study of 100 suicides in 1974 found that 40% had visited their family doctor in the week before they died and over 70% in the previous 3 months. In most cases, the doctors had recognized that the patient was psychologically disturbed because 80% of those who had visited him had received a psychotropic drug or barbiturate. It is important to assess whether a patient is a suicide risk and to enlist other forms of appropriate support for the patient other than prescribing psychotropic drugs.

Discussion may help

Although the doctor may be reluctant to bring up the subject of suicide, suicidal patients are less likely to try to kill themselves when the subject has been discussed openly. Those at risk must be under more surveillance and should be asked to return to the surgery. The Samaritans, a voluntary organization, also offers a 24 hour service which the patient can call if in need of support during the night.

The Mental Health Act

This Act is the basis of today's services for the mentally ill and handicapped and its underlying principle is that mentally disordered people should be treated as far as possible in the same way as someone who is physically ill. Voluntary treatment is encouraged and community care should, where possible, take the place of long periods in hospital.

Compulsory procedures

Occasions arise, however, when a person becomes so disordered and unstable that it is necessary to override his wishes if he refuses hospital treatment. Compulsion must, however, only be used as a last resort when a patient is considered either dangerous to himself or to others.

The Mental Health Act provides two main and one subsidiary compulsory procedures:

The different sections in the Act

(1) Section 25 – detention for a limited period of observation.

(2) Section 26 – detention for a longer period of treatment.

(3) Section 29 – detention for a very short period of observation in an emergency.

It applies to those with mental illnesses, psychopathic disorders, and mental subnormality.

Normally, all patients should have the benefit of two medical opinions before being detained. One of the medical opinions must be from a doctor approved as having specialized knowledge on the subject. The doctor is 'approved' for this purpose by the local health authority. Only in an emergency is it permissible to act on one medical recommendation.

For the purposes of observation (S.25) and observation in an emergency (S.29), the doctor has only to give his opinion that the patient is suffering from a mental disorder, without naming the particular form of disorder and without giving detailed reasons for reaching the conclusion. For the purposes of treatment under S.26, he must name the particular form of disorder *and* also set out reasons for reaching that decision. The two doctors must agree on their conclusions. The recommendations

The recom-
mendations

must always confirm (1) that compulsory admission is necessary either 'in the interests of (the patient's) own health or safety' or for 'the protection of other persons'; (2) that informal admission or other means of dealing with the situation are not appropriate and why; and (3) in an emergency, that the normal procedure would 'involve undesirable delay'.

The medical recommendations form the basis on which an Application for Admission is made to the hospital named. This Application must be made either by the nearest relative (in an emergency any relative) or by an approved social worker in the

The role of the
social worker

local authority social services department. The social worker can, if necessary, override the relative for the purposes of admission for observation, under S.25 and S.29, but cannot do so in the case of admission for treatment under S.26, except with the approval of the county court. It is often preferable if the application is made by a social worker as relatives often find it difficult to sign for the compulsory detention of a member of their family.

The rates of compulsory and emergency admissions varies widely between regions, suggesting that administrative

Rights of
appeal

practices rather than severity of illness are involved. However, patients can appeal against Compulsory Orders to the Mental Health Review Tribunal.

Treatment of mental illness

Broadly speaking, there are three principal modes of treatment open to the general practitioner:

(1)   The psychological, including the behavioural.

(2) Those procedures aimed at modifying the social environment.

(3) The pharmacological.

Psychological methods of treatment

The common mixed affective disorders can impose considerable emotional demands on the general practitioner. At one extreme, the doctor may be expected to share the patient's intense distress and deal with intractable life situations and, on the other, he may have to endure displays of hostility or deal with a number of trivial complaints. These consultations may engender feelings of helplessness, despair or exasperation. However, the doctor can give an enormous amount of help through being sympathetic, giving reassurance, showing interest, respect and avoiding criticism.

Emotional demands on the GP

When a patient fails to disclose his problems and anxieties directly, the doctor has to be sensitive and receptive to all that the patient says to try and find out what the problems are. Patients may only find it possible to reveal their fears and feelings when the doctor is warm, sympathetic, and when he is accepting without showing strong moral judgement.

Need to be sensitive and receptive

Counsellors or therapists whose interventions have shown beneficial effects beyond that observed in equivalent control groups tend to have a number of specific attributes or traits. These characteristics may be described as:

Attributes of therapists who are effective

(1) Genuineness or authenticity, or of 'being themselves'.

(2) Non-possessive warmth – the attitude of a caring, friendly and concerned approach.

(3) Accurate, empathy, the capacity to 'feel with the patient' so that the patient 'feels understood'.

Thus, a patient who is received kindly, who is listened to with patience and consideration, who is not condemned or overtly criticized for his role, will be able to obtain emotional relief by talking about his problems. This may diminish his anxieties so that he is able to perceive events more clearly and manage his life more effectively. Treating a patient with respect will also add to his feelings of his own worth and dignity.

Emotional relief by talking

A patient may also need help in explaining and clarifying what are the major features of his difficulty and the specific needs for which he wants help. It may be helpful to focus on

Need to clarify situation

these key issues and to distinguish which is the most pressing. Sometimes it is beneficial to discuss the advantages and disadvantages of several possible courses of action in order to make a decision easier, the patient arriving at a clearer view of what he wants to do. Alternatively, it may be possible to set the patient a number of simple behavioural goals or to discuss with the patient the specific ways in which he would like to change his situation.

Set behavioural goals

As well as treating the patient himself, the doctor can refer the patient on to a number of agencies for counselling help. As with other problems, it is often better if the patient is not referred immediately on presenting a problem as this can lead to the patient feeling very rejected. This may not only have an effect on the future doctor–patient relationship but can also lead to the patient refusing to take his problem elsewhere, fearing another rejection.

Referral to other agencies

The agency which will be most helpful to the patient will depend in part on the patient's particular problem. A young mother may find the involvement of a health visitor as the most helpful while someone with a marital problem may be helped by a marriage guidance counsellor. Alternatively, a psychiatrist, psychologist, social worker or priest may be willing to help. Many voluntary organizations offer counselling services and self-help groups may be particularly valuable for some problem areas. Many parts of the country have services specifically for young people in difficulties. In addition, the British Association for Counselling has details of agencies who offer therapy, counselling and support.

Agencies who can help

Voluntary agencies

Behaviour methods

The methods have been shown to be particularly helpful in the management of anxiety, phobias and obsessional states. These techniques includes desensitization, flooding and modelling. The former two procedures employ the principles of confronting the patient with the stimuli that upset him until he get used to them. In modelling, the therapist carries out the required behaviours and gets the patient to copy him. Modelling can be used to reduce social anxieties by training the patient in social skills. Techniques to modify behaviour can also be helpful to adults with relationship difficulties or with children.

Behaviour therapy

Behavioural techniques are used by many psychiatrists but it is one of the major methods of treatment used by clinical

Clinical psychologists

psychologists. The psychology department of the local psychiatric hospital may be willing to take referrals of neurotic patients, especially those suffering from phobias, anxieties or obsessions. Many general practices operate schemes whereby clinical psychologists are attached. In addition, experienced social workers with an interest in behaviour therapy can be of help.

There are also a number of voluntary organizations such as the Phobics Society which can be of benefit to patients.

Social methods of treatment

The close association between psychiatric and social morbidity underlines the need to change or improve the patient's social environment. Patients can be referred to the local authority social services department for help with their social problems. When social workers have been attached to general practices, one of their major roles has involved tackling the social problems of patients suffering from psychiatric ill health.

The role of the social worker

Many of the social problems of psychiatric patients, such as marital difficulties, housing and financial problems, are dealt with elsewhere. The remainder of this section will concentrate on the social needs of the more chronically ill and disabled, including the psychotic.

The strain on the family

Living with schizophrenia

Relatives of schizophrenics often describe one of two major problems, both of which are distressing and difficult to live with. Patients may either be withdrawn and lead almost completely solitary lives or they may be excessively active, often behaving in a socially embarrassing way. Relatives may have to endure threats of violence, suicidal attempts or sexually unusual behaviour.

Difficulties encountered by relatives

Expressed emotion

Recent evidence suggests that schizophrenic patients living with highly critical or overinvolved relatives have higher relapse rates than those living alone, in hostel accommodation or in a family rated low on expressed emotion. The evidence suggests that relatives of discharged schizophrenics need to treat the patients in a calm and supportive manner. Relatives may need help in order to learn to cope and coexist with the

Aim to lower
relative's
expectations
of behaviour

afflicted patient's behaviour. It is often better if the relatives leave the patient alone during troublesome periods as well as lower their expectations of how the patients should behave.

Hostel
accommo-
dation

Schizophrenics discharged to highly critical or overinvolved families may do better if transferred to hostel accommodation. Alternatively, it may be helpful if the patient spends much of his time away from home, either in a day centre or a social club. If this is not possible, it may be better if the afflicted patient spends some time in another room away from his relatives.

Other major illnesses

The other major illnesses equally pose a strain on the family. If they involve periods of hospitalization, the individual concerned and relatives have to cope with the after-effects of illness, the possibilities of relapse, continuous medication and the picking up of the threads of a normal life again. Relatives of patients suffering from manic depression will have to cope with extremes of emotion, suicide attempts, withdrawal and misery and then periods of mania and the financial and social problems that often accompany this.

Considerable
long-term
strain on
relatives

Hard work
involved

The elderly person with dementia or paranoia will require skilful handling, patience and often much physical hard work in dressing, feeding, etc. In addition, the relatives of the elderly person may be far from young themselves. In elderly couples, the non-afflicted spouse may find it almost impossible to cope but is unable to consider any alternative form of care.

Day and short-
term care

It is, therefore, not surprising that most relatives experience anxiety, depression and guilt as well as anger. The doctor can help by offering support, advice and sympathy as well as by mobilizing as many services as possible. Day care may enable relatives to carry on with their work, short-term care can also give them a chance of a holiday.

Services for the mentally ill

Lack of
community
provision

Although, since 1959, there has been substantial decline in the number of patients resident in mental hospitals, there is still little in the way of provision for their care in the community. In 1971, 40% of local authorities had no hostel provision, two thirds had no day centres and 60% had no·group houses or other subsidized living arrangements. Although voluntary

107

organizations offer additional provision there is a considerable degree of unmet need in this group. This not only means that the families of patients have to cope with the extra burden but that many patients relapse or become chronically disabled because of the lack of day or suitable residential facilities.

Services for the handi-capped

In theory, however, the full range of services for the physic-ally handicapped and disabled is available to those suffering from mental illness or handicap, including the provision of home helps and meals-on-wheels. The mentally ill and handi-capped may also be eligible for a bus pass entitling them to free travel or reduced fares.

Day care facilities

Some of the major problems of the mentally ill are social isolation, loneliness and a lack of daytime activity. Day services can reduce these problems and also relieve family strains. Day services are provided through the local area health authorities, local social services departments and voluntary organizations.

Local authority day centres

The number of local authority day centres available for the mentally ill will depend very much on the locality. These centres usually provide social, educational and recreational activities and sometimes light industrial work. Some day centres run a rehabilitation programme for those wishing to return to work. Referral to these day centres is usually through a social worker in the social services department.

Day hospitals

The largest providers of day services are the area health authorities who run day hospitals. The aim of these day hospitals is to keep patients out of hospital, to assess, rehabili-tate and treat. The orientation is usually slightly different to that of the day centre with an emphasis on treatment, possibly including individual and group therapy. Patients are often discharged from hospital to these day hospitals but some hospitals also take patients on a preventive basis before they become so ill that they have to be admitted into hospital.

Social clubs

Some hospitals, local authorities and voluntary bodies also run social clubs, patients meeting for a couple of hours during the day or evening, mainly for social and recreational activities. As these clubs are run by a number of different organizations, such as local MIND groups or churches, details can be obtained from the social services department, the Citizens' Advice Bureaux or the local MIND branch.

Housing difficulties and residential care

There is much evidence to show that hospitals are undertaking a burden of residential care for mentally ill and handicapped people who should be living in the community. Many of those in hospital have no home to go to or relatives willing to care for them. As with the elderly and physically handicapped, a major issue is the transfer of patients from one type of facility to another.

Housing association

Those individuals who can manage to look after themselves but who cannot find housing on the open market may find that a housing association will help. The social services department should have details of those associations most likely to help.

Group homes

Patients who need some supervision can be considered for a place in a group home or a halfway house. These are run by psychiatric hospitals, social services departments and voluntary organizations. In group homes, the inhabitants share a number of communal facilities, thus reducing isolation. A social worker or nurse usually supervises. In halfway homes, patients are accommodated on a temporary basis when they learn to adjust to independent living.

Halfway houses

Hostels or boarding-out schemes

Those needing more supervision may find a place in a hostel or be be boarded out with a landlady who supervises and cooks or with a family. The Mental After Care Association also provides a number of hostels with permanent accommodation.

Advice and assistance can be obtained from the social services department, the psychiatric social worker in the local hospital or a branch of MIND.

The mentally handicapped

In 1977, the DHSS estimated that there were 120 000 people in England and Wales who were severly mentally handicapped, of whom 50 000 were children. Medical advances over the last 20 years have resulted in a much longer life expectancy for many types of mental handicaps. However, only a small proportion need constant nursing care and medical supervision, the majority can live with their families or in residential care.

Extent of the problem

There has been a growing recognition that the mentally handicapped have the same rights and needs as the rest of society, including the right to live as full a life as possible. The mentally disordered and handicapped, however, tend to bear a stigma. Thus, many of the handicapped and their relatives

Stigma

restrict their contacts with others to avoid being rejected or shunned.

Emotional and behaviour problems

The severe problems and emotional trauma experienced by the parents of the mentally handicapped are very similar to those suffered by parents with physically disabled children. These are discussed in an earlier chapter on the physically disabled (pp. 80–82).

Behaviour problems

Many handicapped children also exhibit behaviour problems. The doctor can be of help by giving advice on management and the health visitor or social worker may also be involved. Often parents are overindulgent and do too much for the child. In these cases, the parents should be encouraged to allow the child more independence.

Clinical or educational psychologists

Referral to a psychologist in the local psychiatric or mental subnormality hospital can also be helpful in order to obtain a detailed assessment of the child's functioning and capability. Psychologists attached to hospitals or child guidance clinics can help if the child is exhibiting disturbed behaviour as behaviour therapy can often produce good results.

Behaviour therapy

Counselling

Social workers can offer counselling to the mentally handicapped person and his family, although this type of work is unfortunately often given low priority in the social services department. Mentally handicapped adults may need counselling help in their own right, many are unhappy with problems at work, loneliness and sexual frustrations. Usually, much more help can be offered by a voluntary organization such as MENCAP who can offer help and support to the mentally handicapped child, adult or family.

Voluntary organizations

Services for the mentally handicapped

Mentally handicapped people may have a variety of physical handicaps and difficulties, they may be blind, deaf, incontinent, unable to walk or subject to fits. They are thus eligible for the full range of local authority and local area health provision for the disabled (p. 75).

Eligibility for the provision for the disabled

Laundry services

The local area health authorities may provide laundry services, waterproof sheets, pads and plastic pants for the incontinent, wheelchairs and aids for those who have little mobility.

The local authority social services department provides

Aids and
adaptations

Short-term
care

Speech
therapists and
physio-
therapists

domiciliary laundry services as well as aids and adaptations to the home. These aids can help a variety of tasks including mobility, dressing, personal hygiene and feeding. Arrangements can also be made for short-term care of the mentally handicapped child or adult. This can give the relatives a break, often preventing a crisis occurring. Local authorities can also provide meals-on-wheels or a home help service to mentally handicapped adults on their own or more rarely to families.

Mentally handicapped children or adults may also benefit from referral to a speech therapist or a physiotherapist to aid movement.

Educational and occupation provision

Education

The under fives may be accepted in a preschool playgroup, day nursery or nursery school, often mixing with non-handicapped children. Details of facilities are available from the social services department. After 5, the education of the mentally handicapped becomes the responsibility of the local education authority which provides special schools. Any problems at school are thus dealt with by the education authorities or the education welfare service.

Adult training
centres

After 16, the social services department again takes over the responsibility of the mentally handicapped for education and occupation. It provides adult training centres, where the trainees have lessons on home making, shopping, food preparing, personal hygiene, the use of money and public transport. In addition, a variety of occupations and tasks may be given, usually including light industrial work such as packing, sewing or sorting. In 1973, some 31 000 mentally handicapped adults received training in England and Wales and 3200 in Scotland.

Other
facilities for
the disabled

The mentally handicapped adult can also use the services of the Disablement Resettlement Officer, rehabilitation centres for the disabled, Remploy and sheltered workshops. However, in practice, few mentally handicapped adults attend these other work centres or leave the training centres for employment in the open market. Many are capable of more complex work but lack of opportunities and facilities forces many to fail to achieve their full working potential.

Problems with residential care

Although the majority of mentally handicapped live with their families, alternative residential accommodation is necessary

111

The need for residential provision

for almost all severely retarded people at some time in their lives. Mentally handicapped adults may be received into care when their parents become old or die and younger children may need long-term care, especially if their parents reject them or cannot cope with their physical or behavioural problems.

Different schemes

Although local authorities and voluntary organizations provide residential accommodation, places are limited. There are a number of different facilities, group homes, boarding-out schemes and 'foster' parents. There are also residential homes for the more severely disabled child and adult. Most residential homes are small, the maximum is normally 24 for adults, 20 for children.

Few places available

There are, however, few supervised places for adults. Generally, the mentally handicapped are forced to be more dependent on others than is necessary. Hospital residents are often waiting for hostel places while hostel residents are waiting to move out to less sheltered housing. There is a great need to increase unstaffed homes including group homes.

Social services department

Details of long-term care facilities are available from the social services department. Referral will usually result in a social worker visiting the patient or family to assess the situation. Alternatively, voluntary organizations may be able to assist. For example, one voluntary organization 'Parents for Children' specializes in finding foster homes for hard to place children.

Social activities and voluntary organizations

The voluntary organizations play a major role in providing services, social activities and emotional support to the mentally handicapped and their families. They arrange outings, babysitting services, sporting activities such as swimming and riding, parties and holidays with transport provided by volunteers. Parents of handicapped children or adults can benefit greatly from involvement in a local branch of one of those voluntary organizations, receiving and giving help to parents in a similar position to themselves.

Many activities arranged

Trusteeship scheme

There are also a number of schemes to help handicapped adults living with ageing parents. Parents can join a trusteeship scheme (run by MENCAP) by paying a lump sum, by making a bequest in their will or by an insurance policy. When the parents die, a welfare visitor comes regularly to see the mentally handicapped adult and sort out his affairs as well as remember him on his birthday and at Christmas.

Financial problems of the mentally ill and handicapped

Financial
difficulties are
common

Financial problems are common, since having a mentally disabled child or adult in the family involves extra expenditure on items such as transport, clothing and heating. There is also likely to be loss of earnings.

Allowances
and financial
help available

The mentally disabled are entitled to the same range of benefits as the physically handicapped. Those with mentally handicapped children are eligible for the benefits available to all families such as family allowance or family income supplement (if appropriate) as well as attendance, mobility and invalid care allowance. Attendance allowance is payable for children of 2 or older who need substantially more care or supervision than a non-disabled child of the same age or sex. Mobility allowance is payable to children over 5 who are unable or virtually unable to walk. Families may also receive considerable help from the Family Fund or from voluntary organizations.

Adults
eligible for
supple-
mentary
benefit

Mentally handicapped or mentally ill adults are eligible for the non-contributory invalidity pension or supplementary benefit. Patients with a contribution record may also be eligible for sickness benefit or invalidity benefit. Those on supplementary benefit can receive additional payments, where appropriate, for heating, laundry, heavy wear and tear of clothing, diet and fares to the hospital. The Citizens' Advice Bureau services department should be able to advise and help. (Fuller details of these allowances are included in Chapter 6.)

Alcohol problems

Extent of the
problem

Britain is a society in which alcoholic beverages are readily available in High Street supermarkets and off-licences, in which public houses are regarded as convenient places to meet with friends, and where it is unusual for an adult to be totally abstinent. While alcohol consumption is steadily increasing, so is the proportion of the population suffering physical and social damage from drinking. Excessive drinking is claimed to be the fourth major health hazard in Great Britain.

Sharp
increase
among women

This increase in problems due to drinking is particularly great among women who are also more likely to conceal their drinking habits. In 1977, nearly one quarter of diagnosed alcoholics were women and there was a substantial increase in the number of women referred to helping agencies.

Factors affecting susceptibility

Risk factors

High risk
occupation

Women are more likely than men to develop severe alcohol-related illnesses and recent studies suggest that a genetic element may also increase susceptibility. The nature of a person's work is often an influential factor in determining whether someone will drink excessively with high risk occupations including journalism, the catering industry, the Merchant Navy and the medical profession. Isolated or unsupervised jobs, where alcohol is readily accessible and where there are strong pressures among fellow workers to drink are those occupations where individuals are most at risk.

Physical disorders and psychological problems

Physical
illnesses

Alcoholics have a high death rate from accidents, poisoning, violence and from diseases of the circulatory, respiratory and digestive systems. Heavy drinking in pregnancy may bring about fetal and neonatal abnormalities and low birth weight.

Resulting
changes

As the person becomes more dependent on alcohol, his personality may start to change. He may become irritable or anxious when a drink is needed and when drunk can be violent, quarrelsome or morose.

Guilt and
remorse

After a period of excessive drinking, the person is likely to be guilty and full of remorse. He may promise never to drink again or promise to behave better at home or at work. These promises are not likely to be kept and the drinker may be considered to be untrustworthy or irresponsible. The problem drinker may also tell lies about his whereabouts or his drinking habits to avoid arguments with his family. As he becomes more dependent physically, his drinking will become more uncontrollable, making him more anxious and therefore more likely to drink. Suicide is a common occurrence; 8% of those with serious alcohol problems commit suicide.

Lies to avoid
recrimination

Suicide

May cause or
exacerbate
social
problems

These psychological problems and physical ill health will cause social problems or exacerbate those already present. A job may be lost by the individual failing to appear at work due to withdrawal symptoms. Difficult behaviour may cause the spouse to seek a separation or divorce.

Treatment

Early
recognition

Alcohol problems frequently remain hidden in spite of attendance at surgeries and outpatient clinics. The doctor may not

114

link alcohol overuse to the medical, social or psychological problems presented and the patient may feel too full of shame to admit it. The patient's use of alcohol needs to be explored as active, early intervention is vital.

Assessment of drinking habits

Once the doctor has full details of the drinking pattern, some estimate can be made of the seriousness of the dependence. The doctor also needs to assess the patient's capacity for change and the social pressures which make a reduction in drinking difficult.

Motivation to change

In order to change his habits, the patients needs to accept he had a problem and be motivated to overcome some of the difficulties he will have to face. Capacity to change will also

Support from family

depend on the support available from his family and others and his ability to find alternative ways of coping with stress and to occupy his time.

Combination of realism and optimism

The doctor needs to be realistic about the changes that can take place but at the same time optimistic. It is important not to reinforce any punitive or despairing view of alcohol problems. It is still a commonly held view that most people with these problems are unlikely to change and a pessimistic position may be taken which is unhelpful to the patient. Although the patient needs information about the physical

Not to overwhelm

damage which alcohol causes, it is important not to overwhelm the patient which may make him more resistant to asking for help.

Focus of interventions

While brief intensive intervention is sufficient for some patients, those with a chronic problems may need long-term help. Interventions should be focused towards (1) achieving control of alcohol use, through abstinence or reduced intake, (2) in helping the patient to develop new sources of satisfaction and ways of handling stress, and (3) supporting and helping the family to cope. The family may need help in its own right but it also plays a key role in producing change.

With less severe cases, general practitioners can often provide all the necessary medical care and referral to specialist facilities may not be necessary. A social worker or community psychiatric nurse can be involved in treatment or in helping with social problems.

Day care

Some patients can be helped without admission into hospital by day care facilities. These can be provided by hospital treatment units or the social services department and include day shelters, workshops and training centres. Some of these are for a wide range of patients rather than for alcoholics only.

In addition, many people with drinking problems are helped

115

Alcoholics
Anonymous

by the voluntary agencies in this field, particularly Alcoholics Anonymous which is based on the 'self-help' principle. Details are in Appendix 6.

Residential care

Hospital facilities

There are approximately 36 specialist treatment units in Britain. Some are within psychiatric hospitals, others are within psychiatric departments of district general hospitals.

Treatment in hospital

Most units have a planned programme of treatment which includes a range of group and individual activities. Some units include programmes designed to teach moderate drinking but usually abstinence is stressed. Individual counselling and groupwork may be the responsibility of psychiatrist, nurse, social worker, psychologist or occupational therapist. These units usually maintain contact with each individual after the initial intensive period of treatment which may involve detoxication, drying out, drug treatment or aversion therapy. Aftercare may be carried out in collaboration with other community based services such as social workers.

In those regions without specialist units, the general psychiatric service will offer help. In 1975, 7% of all admissions to the general psychiatry services of England and Wales had a diagnosis of alcoholism.

Social problems associated with excessive drinking

Problems with interpersonal relationships

Marital problems

The most frequent social problems for the overuser of alcohol are in his personal relationships. The marital partner is likely to experience fewer of the satisfactions expected from marriage and at the same time will have to take over the role for which the drinking spouse previously took responsibility. For example, a wife may have to work to pay the bills, alternatively the husband may have to look after the children and do the housework. In addition, drinking frequently precedes violence between spouses, and it may commonly precede child abuse. It is obviously a factor in marital disharmony and may be the principal cause of disagreement, separation and divorce.

Effects of separation and divorce

Marital breakdown usually increases the problem of the alcohol abuser. When the marriage ends, the person often finds it difficult to maintain a secure and comfortable home, and

116

becomes less motivated to maintain his personal appearance, to keep to a balanced diet or to hold down a job. Research studies suggest that the problem drinker who has lost his (or her) spouse is less likely to maintain sobriety after treatment than those whose marriages remain intact.

Effects on children
Children are likely to be particularly vulnerable to harm in a family where one or both parents are drinking excessively. Young children, bewildered and frightened by what is happening, may demonstrate a wide range of disturbed and disturbing behaviour. Older children, with a clearer understanding of the cause of family difficulties, may experience considerable distress and feel forced to take responsibility for one or both parents. The premature maturity that is imposed on such children may seriously reduce the energy available for the normal and necessary activities of childhood and adolescence.

These problems may be helped by a number of agencies as well as by the doctor, including community psychiatric nurses, marriage guidance workers, social workers and voluntary agencies specific to this area.

Financial and legal problems

Debts and employment difficulties
Financial difficulties are common as money formerly allocated to the payment of bills or rent may be spent on drink. Thus, eviction or gas or electricity disconnections may occur. Employment difficulties caused by drinking may exacerbate the situation.

Court appearance

The role of other agencies
Court appearances may also occur, either due to the accumulating debts or criminal offences, such as being drunk and disorderly, driving and drinking, or violent offences. Probation officers may be able to help as well as the social services department. The disablement resettlement officer will also help with the employment problems of the alcoholic.

Withdrawal and isolation

Social deterioration
Someone preoccupied with drinking is likely to develop a life style different from that of his friends and family. He may increasingly drink by himself, sometimes secretly, thus increasing his social isolation. He may also be at risk of social deterioration, losing interest in his appearance or personal hygiene and becoming nocturnally incontinent. A critical and

117

rejecting spouse may make matters worse and start the alcoholic off on a downward spiral. Voluntary agencies may be able to offer the most help and support with these difficulties.

The homeless alcoholic

There are a number of facilities for alcoholics who are homeless or who have no family willing to help them. Sheltered accommodation may be available to those who require little supervision and assistance (details from the social services department).

A number of agencies run night shelters and houses, such as the Cyrenians and the Salvation Army. They provide overnight shelter, food and warmth and in some cases the staff try to help Facilities the clients to change their way of life. Special hostel facilities available have also been developed for those trying to move away from the 'Skid Row' way of life and for people who need a period of residential care as a halfway stage between hospital and an independent life. These hostels vary considerably in the methods of treatment given, some emphasize friendship or informal support, others arrange a formal rehabilitation programme.

Drug addiction

Many of the problems of the alcoholic are similar to those of the drug addict and there is considerable overlap between those who drink alcohol excessively and those who abuse drugs. The drug addict is dependent physically and psychologically on drugs. Fortunately, most people take drugs in a responsible manner, normally under medical supervision. However, with some drugs there is always a risk of developing dependency.

The risk of addiction is higher with certain 'hard' drugs such as heroin and cocaine and the physical and social deterioration accompanying addiction gives rise to much social concern. The drug taker can become seriously ill through an overdose or by an unhygienic administration. He can behave irresponsibly while under the influence of the drug. He can neglect himself Social and his family, withdrawing from society, avoiding all problems of responsibilities and losing his job. In addition, he many the addict become part of a drug subculture where his friends and contacts are all involved in drug taking and drug pushing. This

118

may lead him into committing criminal offences in order to have enough money to buy more supplies of the drug.

Registration   In Great Britain, it is possible for addicts to become registered. Once registered, they can be treated and receive prescriptions for their drugs legitimately. This has been found to cut down on the drug addict's criminal activities which were undertaken to obtain supplies of drugs.

Treatment

As with alcoholism, early detection of individuals susceptible to becoming addicts is very important. Doctors have to notify the Home Office of any patient they consider is addicted to a dangerous drug. Treatment is usually voluntary but an addict can be compulsorily admitted under the Mental Health Act when he presents a danger to himself or others.

Drug dependence units   There are approximately 79 drug dependence units in the United Kingdom. These clinics treat addicts as inpatients and outpatients. Treatment is also available in the general psychiatric hospitals.

Other help available   As with alcoholism, treatment usually involves a period of detoxication followed by rehabilitation, aiming to help the addict to give up the dependency. Rehabilitation may involve individual or group psychotherapy or behaviour therapy. While the disablement resettlement officer may help with employment, the social worker may be able to help with some of the addict's other social problems or housing. Unfortunately, there is very little provision for rehabilitation of addicts into the community, especially outside London. Voluntary organizations, such as RELEASE, give all types of help to the drug addict (see Appendix 6 for address) and have the latest information on other helping agencies.

Many ex-addicts return to drug-taking after treatment. Once discharged, they often return to the same environment as before and mix with their old friends who are also taking drugs. Breaking the habit may be only possible when new friends are made and new activities and pastimes taken up.

Summary of the services and help available

In addition to the services listed below, there are many services provided by psychiatric hospitals. These include day hospitals, day care, social clubs and residential provisions including group homes.

119

Problems in social care

Agency	Type of help
Local authority social services department	Social work assistance in compulsory admissions (24 hour emergency service normally available)
	Social work counselling and advice to mentally ill, mentally handicapped and their families
	Short-term care
	Residential facilities
	Recreational facilities, social clubs
	Day care, including the mentally handicapped under 5 or after leaving school (adult training centres)
	Laundry services for the mentally handicapped
	Financial assistance (through the Family Fund or charities)
	Sheltered employment and workshops

In addition, the mentally ill and disabled are entitled to the same services as the physically handicapped such as meals-on-wheels, bus passes, etc.

Health visitor	Support, supervision and counselling to the mentally ill and handicapped and their families
	Help with the behaviour problems of the handicapped
Community psychiatric nurse	Support and therapy for the more severely psychiatrically ill in the community, including giving injections
Probation service	Support and help for the alcoholic or mentally ill offender
Clinical psychologist	Therapy and assessment for the mentally ill and handicapped, including behaviour therapy

Summary of services and help available   (continued)

Local education authority

Specialized schooling

Help of the education welfare officer

Department of local employment
(employment office)

The help of the disablement resettlement officer and sheltered workshops,
Remploy, etc.

Local offices of the Department of
Health and Social Security

Financial help including the following
benefits:
national insurance invalidity
pension
non-contributory invalidity pension
attendance allowance
invalid care allowance
mobility allowance
supplementary benefit

Voluntary agencies

Emotional support to patient and
family

Social and leisure activities

Babysitting services

Transport

Holidays

Schools

Sheltered workshops

Trusteeship scheme

Financial help

Specialized housing and residential
homes (including housing associations)

Housing problems

This chapter deals with the housing difficulties of all age groups including families, single people and the elderly. Details on the specialized accommodation available for the elderly, physically and mentally disabled are covered under the relevant chapters.

General housing difficulties

Housing standards have generally improved over the last 30 years with fewer slums and less overcrowding. However, there still a high proportion of people who have housing problems or who are dissatisfied with their housing. Finding a suitable home at a reasonable price is probably one of the commonest problems faced by individuals and families.

One of the commonest problems

First, there is a chronic shortage of housing in many areas of the country. Although there is approximately the same number of 'dwellings' as there are 'households' in Great Britain, there are too many houses in some places and too few in others, such as the major cities. This means that there are still individuals and families who are homeless or live in overcrowded conditions.

Shortage of housing

Secondly, much of our housing stock is unsuitable or inadequate. Only a small proportion of housing is of recent construction; one quarter of our houses is over 80 years old. This, together with the high cost of maintenance, means that much accommodation is in a poor state of repair or lacks basic amenities. Surveys indicate that approximately 3 million (one

Inadequacy of housing

sixth of the housing stock) lack these amenities or are in disrepair. In 1973, more than one in ten households had only an outside lavatory and almost as many had no bathroom. However, even with more modern buildings, there are still problems. For example, tower blocks have been found to be unsuitable for large proportions of the population, such as those with young children or the elderly, while people housed on the new estates often complain of the lack of community spirit.

The high cost of living

Thirdly, there are problems linked with financial difficulties. Although housing is a basic human need, it differs from others in that it is a very expensive commodity, costing much to build and maintain. Very few people can afford to buy their property outright and others, especially those with large families or with a low income, cannot afford to rent suitable accommodation. The scarcity of adequate housing in many areas make matters worse by increasing the costs of buying and renting. Thus, many families and individuals have to live in inadequate or overcrowded conditions because they cannot afford anything else. The high costs of housing have been recognized by successive governments in recent years who have set up a number of schemes to give financial assistance to all sections of the housing market.

Security of tenure

Fourthly, there are problems related to security of tenure, particularly for those who rent accommodation. This can cause much anxiety and worry, although the recent rent acts have given much more security to tenants.

Resulting health difficulties

It is, therefore, not surprising that housing difficulties are one of the commonest social problems presented to general practitioners. Poor housing conditions can lead to a number of health problems as well as psychological and social difficulties. Marital dysfunction or breakdown and child neglect can be due, at least in part, to the strain of living in poor conditions or the fear of eviction. Depression and anxiety can result from the social isolation found on the newer estates or from the problems of living in a tower block.

Type of accommodation and financial assistance available

There are many types of housing tenure, owner occupied, council housing and renting from a landlord or housing association. By 1975, over half of all householders were owner-occupiers, a third had council accommodation and less than a fifth rented privately from a landlord. This last type of accommodation has diminished considerably in recent years, partly due to the various acts of Parliament making renting out privately less profitable for the landlord.

Owner-occupation

Owning one's home has many advantages, there is greater security and it is a means of investment and saving. Most homes are bought and sold on the open market, using estate agents or advertising in the local newspapers. Many local authorities also sell properties (details from the town hall) and in many areas, council tenants can buy their homes, often at a large discount. Another way of buying a home is through a housing association where the ownership of the property is on a co-operative basis. Details can also be obtained from the Citizens' Advice Bureau or the National Federation of Housing Associations.

Places from which a loan can be obtained
Loans for house purchase are available from a number of sources, from building societies, insurance companies, banks and from the local authority. Local authorities specialize as lenders of last resort or older properties, and in lending to those affected by compulsory purchase and to groups with special needs.

Tax relief and schemes to help
Mortgages are normally eligible for tax relief on mortgage repayments. There are some people on low incomes, however, who pay insufficient tax to allow them to obtain the full benefit of tax relief. For those people, the government Option Mortgage Scheme or the Option Mortgage Guarantee scheme might help. The details of both government schemes for helping house purchasers are rather complicated, but explanatory booklets on each of them can be obtained from building societies or Citizens' Advice Bureau.

Mortgage arrears
Owner-occupiers who are unable to meet their mortgage commitments should discuss this with the building society to try and extend the period of the loan. If they are in receipt of supplementary benefit they may be eligible to have the interest element of the mortgage paid by the DHSS, together with any ground rent and rates. Charitable organizations may also be able to help in special circumstances.

Rent rebates
Owner-occupiers are also eligible for a rate rebate if their income is very low. This can be particularly helpful for pensioners with large houses.

125

Local authority housing

The need for council housing

After the First World War, good housing was recognized as a need for which society must accept responsibility. The local authorities were encouraged by subsidies to provide and build accommodation which could be let at a low rent. Thus, large sections of the population who could not afford to buy their own homes or pay high rents could still be housed adequately. The first council houses were designed to replace the slums and house slum dwellers which may explain part of the stigma still attached to living in council accommodation. Council housing has now developed to such an extent that the local authorities are now responsible for housing 20 million people.

Those who are helped

The housing waiting list

Individuals and families are housed by the council by being on the housing list, by demolition and slum clearance of their old homes, through exchanges or transfer and for medical reasons. The selection of tenants for housing rests with the local housing authority which maintains a housing list, ensuring that accommodation goes to those whose need is most urgent. Frequently, applicants are allocated houses on a 'points' system, points being assessed according to size of family, length of residence, degree of overcrowding, etc. Local authorities vary considerably in how much notice they take of a

Medical grounds

doctor's letter asking for urgent consideration of a patient on health grounds. The length of waiting lists varies from authority to authority, but Shelter, a voluntary organization, estimated, from a survey carried out in July 1977, that nationally there are over one million households on housing waiting lists.

Transfer on death of tenant

When the family members responsible for payments dies, the tenancy can sometimes be transferred to another member of the family. However, this is usually a process where no general procedure is followed and it varies between authorities.

Financial help including rent and rate rebates

'Reasonable' rents

Local authorities are required to charge their tenants 'reasonable' rents without making a profit. Local authorities also operate schemes for granting rent rebates to council tenants and rent allowances to private tenants. Tenants or owner-occupiers may also get rebate from their rates. Enquiries should be made to the Rent Rebate Allowance Officer in the Town Hall.

The amount of rebate or allowance is computed according to a formula bases on the rent or rates of the accommodation, the

Housing problems

gross income of the tenant, size of the household and the personal circumstances. Income includes earnings plus any benefits except attendance and mobility allowances. People on supplementary benefit are not normally eligible for rent or rate rebates and allowances.

Rent arrears
Council tenants who are in receipt of supplementary benefit and who accrue arrears of rent may be helped by having their rent paid direct to the housing authority by the DHSS. In certain cases the DHSS will also pay an amount towards the arrears. Enquiries should be made to the local DHSS office. Charities may also help in paying off arrears and a social worker from the local authority may be able to assist in contacting suitable organizations.

Housing associations

Enormous growth in this sector
Large charitable trusts such as Peabody and Guinness Trusts have long owned large housing estates. More recently, however, there has been an enormous growth in the voluntary housing movement, and in 1976 there were 250 000 housing association dwellings in England and Wales.

Those groups catered for
The main purpose of housing associations is to provide rented accommodation. Some are charitable trusts, some are registered companies, none are profit-making. Housing associations usually provide rented accommodation for those with small incomes, employees of particular companies, special groups or classes like old people, handicapped people or immigrants. There are also 'self-help' societies which provide collectively owned accommodation on a co-operative or co-partnership basis.

Priority given to groups in need
Housing associations provide a valuable addition to the stock of rented accommodation because of their flexibility and because of the priority they give to groups in special need. Patients can obtain information about these associations from the local Citizens' Advice Bureau, social services department or the National Federation of Housing Associations.

The tenancies are subject to the fair rent system as in council housing. Tenants are eligible for rent and rate rebates.

Privately rented housing

Traditionally, this was the most important section of housing providing 90% of homes at the beginning of the century. It has

127

decline sharply in the postwar years and now provides for about 12% of all households. This type of accommodation has the advantage that people can move fairly easily although there is less security of tenure. However, private rented accommodation at reasonable rent is difficult to find in many areas, especially the large cities.

Financial help available

Tenants of private landlords may be eligible for rent allowances and rate rebates. In addition, tenants are protected from high
rents by the 'fair rent' service. If a tenant considers his rent is too high, he may apply to the rent officer through the town hall (or the rent tribunal office if his landlord lives on the premises). The rent officer determines a fair rent on application by the tenant or landlord. If either object to his assessment, they can appeal to the Rent Assessment Committee. When a rent has been registered (based on the state of repair, age and locality of the property) a tenant cannot legally be required to pay more, apart from increases in rates. The rent is fixed for a period of 2 years unless there are changes such as alterations to the dwelling. A tenant fearful of eviction should be made aware of his tenancy 'rights'. A landlord cannot change the registered rent even when the tenant leaves and another one takes his place.

Tied accommodation

This is when the accommodation is tied to a job and accounts for one million dwellings. The tenant in this type of housing often lacks security as when he loses his job he also loses his accommodation. Recently, however, those working in agriculture have increased security of tenure.

Squatting

This is a term used to describe the action taken when an individual or group occupies empty property to which they have no legal right. Some local authorities have made agreements with groups squatting in their property and will allow the groups limited tenure in return for payment of rates and an agreement to move to another nominated property when required. With
out such agreements, squatting can lead to proceedings in the civil court and in many cases the owners of the property can regain possession quickly. Squatters also run the risk of

prosecution under the laws relating to forcible entry, burglary
and criminal damage. Information on squatting can be obtained
from Shelter or the Special Advisory Service for Squatters.

Homelessness

The number of homeless has steadily grown due to the great
rise in the cost of homes, the decline in the privately rented
sector and the increase in the overall number of households
(earlier marriages, more single-parent families, more elderly).
The homeless are usually young and are either single or have
young families. Those with young children are usually on low
incomes and may have recently separated from their spouse or
been evicted by their landlord. The single homeless are often
migrants, ex-hospital patients, ex-offenders or the unemployed.
In 1976, there were 30 000 homeless people living in local
authority temporary accommodation. However, this figure is an
underestimate of the total number of homeless.

Local authorities have a duty to find accommodation for a
person who becomes homeless without intent and who has
priority need. Priority cases included those who have children
or are pregnant, those who are homeless due to an emergency
or a disaster such as fire or flood and those who are vulnerable
for some reason (including pensioners, the physically and
mentally disabled and battered wives).

A homeless person or family should apply to the housing
department of the local authority. In some cases there is a
special section. Applicants are investigated thoroughly to find
out whether they are homeless, whether this was intentional
and whether they are a priority case. Efforts will be made to
persuade relatives or friends to help. Local authorities do not
house homeless people readily because of their responsibilities
to those on the waiting list and in other situations. Often help
from a social worker, solicitor or law centre may be necessary if
the individual or family is refused accommodation. Sometimes, bed and breakfast accommodation is offered at first or
temporary housing followed by an ordinary council tenancy.

Homeless single people

Most single people would not be considered by the local
authority as in priority need except, for example, a pregnant

woman or a disabled person. There are, however, a number of hostels and lodging houses available to cater for this group. This includes the YMCA, YWCA, the Salvation Army, night shelters provided by the Cyrenians and resettlement units and reception centres run by the DHSS. The social services department can give advice and information on hostels or alternative accommodation for the single homeless. There are a number of addresses of organizations who help the single homeless in Appendix 7.

Problems of unsuitable or substandard housing

In spite of much slum clearance, there are a high proportion of houses still below standard. Many of these are occupied by those on low incomes or the elderly or handicapped. While many people live in overcrowded conditions, others occupy houses or flats too big for them, particularly the elderly whose families have left.

Help for tenants

Certificate of disrepair

Landlords of very substandard rented accommodation can be compelled by the local authority to do the necessary repairs for the health of the occupant. The local authority can issue a certificate of disrepair entitling the tenant to a reduced rent until the repairs are carried out or standard amenities installed.

Multiple occupancy

The local authority can also impose a limit on the number of households or persons who may live in a house and can require that certain amenities such as baths, WCs and fire escapes are increased in houses of multiple accommodation. Although

Fear of eviction

tenants can apply to the local authority (town hall) for help and advice, many do not complain because they are fearful of eviction or harassment by the landlord.

Grants available for repairs

Secure tenants as well as owner-occupiers and landlords are also eligible to claim house renovation grants to improve their property. Improvement grants are discretionary, while intermediate grants are obligatory and are made to provide any basic amenities such as a bath or inside WC which are missing. In certain areas such as 'general improvement areas' grants are easier to obtain and cover a higher percentage of the cost. Applications should be made to the local authority.

Unsuitable council housing

Council transfers

Local authorities vary according to how easy it is to change council accommodation. Patients wishing to transfer can apply

130

to the housing department and may ask for a doctor's letter to support their request. Alternatively, tenants wishing to change accommodation may consider advertising privately in the local papers or newspaper shop.

Other problems

Excessive noise from neighbours or industry

Anyone concerned about excessive noise from neighbours or industry can also seek help from the environmental health inspector in the local authority. If the local authority decide to act, they can serve a notice on the person responsible for the noise and can bring about a prosecution if necessary.

Problems of vermin

The local authority health department can also give advice and information on how to tackle any problems of vermin or infestation. They may also carry out treatment, sometimes free of charge.

Tenancy problems

Housing legislation is very complex and many tenants are ignorant of their rights. They may be evicted or endure harassment from their landlord when they have a right to security of tenure. Tenants with problems should consult the Citizens' Advice Bureau, law centre, rent tribunal office, solicitor or local authority.

Security of tenure

Court Order necessary for eviction

The law on security of tenure depends mainly on whether the landlord and tenant live under the same roof. However, no one can be evicted without a Court Order.

Rent Act security

Tenants of all types of accommodation which are not part of the landlord's home are normally protected by rent act security, including council and housing association tenants. They can be evicted when a Court Order has been made on one or more of the grounds covered by the Rent Act. These include non-payment of rent, conduct which is a nuisance to neighbours, the landlord's reasonable need to use the dwelling as a residence for himself or his family or when the dwelling was originally let on a short-term basis. The landlord can only apply to the court for a Court Order 4 weeks after he has given the tenants a written notice to quit.

131

Problems in social care

Tenancies with a resident landlord

Tenancies with a resident landlord must also be given a written notice to quit by the landlord and allowed 4 weeks in which to do so. If the tenant has not left after 4 weeks, the landlord can apply to the court for a Possession Order but it is only after this Order is obtained that the tenant can be evicted legally. If the letting commenced before November 1980, the tenant can suspend the operation of a notice to quit by applying to the local rent tribunal.

Other tenancy problems

Harassment

Illegal eviction is a criminal offence, as is harassing a tenant with the intention of making him give up his rights to his home. The local authority has specific powers to prosecute for these offences and so any complaints should be made to the local authority concerned.

Rent books

Any landlord who lets residential accommodation on a weekly basis must provide a rent book or other similar document – unless he provides board as well as lodging and the value of the board forms a substantial element of the rent. In addition, the landlord must, on written request of a tenant, supply his name or address. If the landlord is a company, the names and addresses of the directors or the secretary of the company should be given.

132

Summary of services and help available

Agency	*Type of help*
Local authority housing department	Help to the homeless in priority need
	Help to those in need of housing through the housing list (local authorities vary according to the notice they take of medical recommendations)
	Help to those whose houses are due to be demolished
	The opportunity to transfer or exchange council housing (the ease of obtaining a transfer will depend on the area)
	Repairs for council housing
Other local authority departments	Rent rebates to those on low incomes in rented or council accommodation (apply to rent rebate allowance officer in the town hall)
	Rate rebates to those on low incomes who pay rates
	Assessment of a 'fair rent' through the rent officer or the rent tribunal office (the latter to be approached if the landlord lives on the premises)
	Advice on security of tenure (rent officer or rent tribunal office will help)
	Help to those renting very unsuitable or overcrowded housing by prosecuting the landlord
	Help to those being harassed by their landlord (harassment officer)
	Housing renovation grants to improve properties or to install basic amenities (landlords, secure tenants or owner-occupiers may be eligible)

Summary of services and help available (continued)

	Help to stop excessive noise from neighbours or problems with infestations or vermin (the environmental health officer)
Local authority housing aid centres and social services departments (social workers)	Advice and assistance on all aspects of housing, including help to those who consider themselves homeless and who have not been helped by the housing department
Voluntary provision including housing associations	Different types of housing (rented or co-ownership) for those who have difficulties in securing accommodation

Other agencies

Further information and specialist advice on housing problems can be obtained from Citizens' Advice Bureaux, housing aid centres, solicitors and law centres. More specialized organizations are included in Appendix 7.

Financial, employment and legal problems

Financial problems

This chapter covers many of the benefits which may be available to patients. However, some benefits and allowances are described in more detail under the relevant chapter, for example, allowances for the physically disabled are included in the chapter on the handicapped.

Poverty

A basic cause of many personal and social problems is lack of money. Often it is said that people do not need professional help from social workers, just money. Higher child benefits, for example, may reduce certain child care problems while more money for the disabled may help them manage at home more easily.

The poverty line Investigators now base the poverty line on the scale of allowances laid down by the Supplementary Benefits Commission or slightly above. These scales can be regarded as the standards set by society below which no one should normally fall.

The groups in society who are poor In the 1950s and 1960s, surveys showed that approximately between 4 and 12% of the population lived below the supplementary scale. If we include those living on supplementary benefit, those living on or below the poverty line consist mainly of retirement pensioners, full-time workers on low incomes, the unemployed, single-parent families and the sick and disabled. As the numbers of elderly, unemployed and one-parent families steadily increase so does the percentage of people living in poverty.

Financial help

Agencies responsible for financial help
This is available mainly from the Department of Health and Social Security which is the central government authority responsible. Social security legislation applies to Scotland as well as England and Wales. In Northern Ireland, the same benefits apply in general.

Financial help is also available from the social services department and Department of Education in certain circumstances. Voluntary bodies also play a role; there are many organizations and charities which have funds available for families and individuals with particular needs.

Contributory and non-contributory benefits

Cash or kind
Some benefits are paid in cash while others take the form of subsidizing the cost of particular services and goods, for example, free prescriptions or free school meals.

Table 3 shows the range of benefits that are available. Basically, there are two types of benefits, contributory and non-contributory. Rights to the former depend on the membership of the individual (or sometimes the husband) of the national insurance scheme. Contributory benefits include retirement and widow's pensions, sickness, unemployment, invalidity and maternity benefits. The amount of benefit paid is related to the number of national insurance contributions paid into the scheme. In certain cases, contributions of a husband count towards benefits obtainable by a wife. Generally, everyone of working age has to pay national insurance contributions if they earn over a certain amount.

Contributory benefits

Non-contributory benefits
Non-contributory benefits do not depend on these contributions and are payable to all those who meet the conditions of eligibility. These benefits include supplementary benefit, family income supplement and child benefit.

Some benefits are means tested (e.g. supplementary benefit) others are not (e.g. child benefit). Some benefits are also taxable and are added to a family's income for tax purposes while others are not.

136

Table 3 Current benefits

National insurance contributory benefits	*National insurance non-contributory benefits*	*Non-contributory means-tested benefits**
Employment benefit	Old person's pension (over 80)	Supplementary benefit
Sickness benefit	Attendance allowances	Family income supplement
Invalidity benefit	Child benefit	Rent and rate rebate/ allowance
Maternity benefit	Invalid care allowance	Prescription, dental treatment
Retirement pension	Mobility allowance	Appliances and drugs supplied by hospitals
Guardian's allowance	Invalidity pension	
Child's special allowance	War pension	Educational benefits
Death grant		Fares to hospital
Widow's benefits		Free milk and vitamins
Industrial injury benefit		Legal advice/aid

*The benefits are automatic and not means-tested for certain groups in the population

Non-take-up of benefits

Take-up rates Unfortunately, the system of benefits is very complex and many people are unaware of their eligibility to claim for certain benefits. The take-up rates vary widely according to the benefit concerned and for family income supplement and housing allowances, take-up is less than 50%. In 1975, £240 million was considered to be the total of unclaimed supplementary benefits.

The reasons why people do not claim are numerous. Firstly,

Reasons why
people fail to
claim

it may be due to ignorance. For example, many families where one parent works may not realize that they are eligible for a supplement to their income. There is also the great stigma involved in claiming, particularly among groups like the elderly. The leaflets describing benefits are often difficult to understand and the officials involved can often be unhelpful.

Help in filling
up forms

Individuals and families may need much coaxing to get them to apply. If they need help filling up forms, the Citizens' Advice Bureau, a social worker or health visitor may be able to help.

Appeals

Appeals

A claimant can appeal against a decision made regarding a benefit by contacting the local security office. Appeals are first heard by an independent local tribunal and then by a social security commissioner if still not settled.

Obtaining
advice about
appealing

Advice about making an appeal can be obtained from the local Citizens' Advice Bureau or legal advice centre. After the appeal letter has been received, the authorities reconsider the original decision before the case is sent to the tribunal so sometimes the claimant may win without even going to the tribunal. Often claimants do better if they attend the hearing with a professional such as a social worker but they cannot obtain legal aid to be represented legally.

Details of specific benefits

Help if sick

Sickness
benefit

Sickness benefit is paid to people normally employed for the first 6 months in which they are incapable of work, due to illness or disablement. The standard weekly rate is increased according to whether the individual has a wife or other adult dependant and according to the number of children. However, if the wife or other adult dependant is earning over a certain amount, the claimant does not get this supplement. Those over pensionable age who are not retired may claim this benefit up to the age of 70 for a man or 65 for a woman.

Invalidity
pension

After 28 weeks, invalidity pension replaces sickness benefit. Invalidity allowance may be paid in addition. These benefits are generally non-taxable and are increased if there are dependants.

Help if unemployed

Unemploy-
ment benefit

Patients who become unemployed should claim as soon as possible at the local unemployment benefit office. They should also register for work at the local employment office or job centre.

Benefit rates are the same as for sickness benefit and are paid for a period of a year. When a person has left his job voluntarily or has been dismissed for misconduct, unemployment benefit will not be paid for a period of up to 6 weeks. Additional conditions for unemployment benefit apply to a number of groups, such as widows, students, and occupational pensioners over 60, but special leaflets are available from the unemployment benefit office.

Help when pregnant

Maternity
grant

Maternity
allowance

Maternity grant is now payable to all pregnant women and may be claimed from 14 weeks before the expected date of birth to 3 months afterwards. It is non-taxable. Maternity allowance is paid on the mother's contribution record, therefore only working women can claim. It is payable for 18 weeks, starting 11 weeks before the expected week of confinement but only if the mother gives up work during this period. It is non-taxable.

Help for the bereaved

Widow's
benefits

There are three benefits for widows, widow's allowance, widowed mother's allowance and widow's pension. If the husband has died as a result of an industrial injury or accident or prescribed disease, a widow may also be entitled to industrial death benefit.

How to claim

Only the late husband's contribution record counts towards widow's benefits. A claim can be made by completing the certificate issued by the registrar and taking it to a local social security office. All widow's benefits are taxable and cease on remarriage or on living with a man as his wife.

Widow's
allowance and
widowed
mother's
allowance

Widow's allowance is paid for the first 6 months of bereavement. It is payable to a widow over 60 only if she is not eligible for retirement pension. It is increased if there are any other dependants. Widowed mother's allowance is payable to widowed mothers from the end of the 6 month period of the widow's allowance. It is increased according to the number of children.

Widow's pension   Widow's pension is payable after the first 6 months to widows who are over 40 at the time of the husband's death or at the time when they cease to be eligible for the widowed mother's allowance. The amount of pension given depends on the widow's age at bereavement or age at the time widowed mother's allowance ceases.

Death grant   In addition to these benefits, a death grant is payable on the death of a contributor, or certain of his/her dependants. The amount of the grant depends on the age of the person who has died and is not taxable. A certificate issued by the registrar should be sent or taken to the local social security office and a claim made within 6 months of the date of death.

War pensions

War pensions   There are two benefits available, the war disablement pension for those disabled as a result of service in the armed forces, and the war widow's and dependant's pension.

Help for those with children

Child benefit   Child benefit is payable for all children under 16 (or under 19 is still in education) and is tax free. Anyone responsible for a child can claim but normally the mother receives the benefit.

Increase rate for single-parent families   Divorced, separated and single parents may be entitled to an increase in the rate. However, this increase is not payable to anyone living with someone as man and wife or who is in receipt of certain benefits. Single parents who are at work can claim an additional personal allowance against income tax.

Family income supplement   Family income supplement is payable to low income families with at least one child where the head of the family is at work for 30 or more hours a week (24 hours if single-parent family). Single-parent families and the self-employed can also claim.

Family income, supplement may be claimed where the gross income of the head of the household and of his wife falls below a level which depends on the number of children. The amount of benefit is equal to half the difference between the qualifying income and actual income up to a maximum amount.

Automatic entitlement to other benefits   Eligibility for family income supplement automatically entitles families to certain other benefits such as free NHS benefits, free milk and vitamins for expectant mothers and

140

young children, free school meals and refund of hospital fares. Post offices have claim forms and details of family income supplements.

Financial help with schooling

Financial help
As education is compulsory, a number of services are available to help the parents get their children to school and keep them there.

Free travel
Children attending local education authority schools are able to obtain free transport to and from schools if they live more than a certain distance away. Arrangements for this travel are made through the school. Alternatively, the education authority may provide a school bus.

Free school meals
There is normally a charge for school dinner but if the family is managing on a low income or benefits (such as supplementary benefit), the dinners can be free. In addition, some

Help with uniform, clothes and footwear
local education authorities give financial help towards the cost of school uniforms, clothes and shoes, and there is a means test for this. Applications for this and free school meals should be made to the school, education department or education welfare office.

Maintenance grants
When children remain at school after the compulsory school leaving age, maintenance allowances may be paid when the

Help for low income families
family income is low. The amount of grant given will depend on income. Children of low income families may also receive help with the cost of school journeys and visits.

Other benefits and allowances

Families may also be eligible for supplementary benefit (described later in the chapter) or help with housing costs, such as rate or rent rebates.

Other help for low income families
A range of means-tested benefits is available for families or single persons where income lies slightly above supplementary benefit level. Help is given with charges for prescriptions, dentures, dental treatment, glasses, milk and vitamins and fares to hospital for treatment. In some cases all charges are met, on others where the income is slightly higher, part of the cost is met.

Help from the local authority
Local authorities may also assist families financially if it prevents a child being received into care, prevents a child

141

appearing before a juvenile court or allows a child to be discharged from care. Local authorities, however, vary considerably in their willingness to make a payment which may be in cash or in kind.

Guardian's allowance and child's special allowance

A person taking an orphan child into the family can claim a guardian's allowance. Child's special allowance is payable to a divorced mother if her ex-husband dies while he was still contributing to the child's upkeep.

Help for pensioners

Retirement pension

Pensions

This is payable to men and women at the age of 65 for men or 60 for women provided they satisfy the contribution condition and have retired from regular work. When a man reaches 70 or a woman 65, retirement pension is payable whether or not they have retired.

A married woman can get a retirement pension on her husband's contribution when he retires and draws his pension provided she is over 60 or over 65 if working. Men or women who work will lose some of their pension if they earn over a certain amount and it may be wise not to draw one's pension until later if at work.

The very old

Pensioners aged 80 or over receive a little extra. Non-contributory retirement pension may be paid to anyone over 80 if they were not already eligible for national insurance retirement pension.

In recent years, a new pension scheme has been started. Under this scheme, retirement, widow's and invalidity pensions may include an additional pension related to earnings provided the person has not 'contracted out'.

Other benefits

Supplementary benefit

Supplementary benefit is payable to old people who are not eligible for a retirement pension. However, those living on retirement pensions should also check to see whether they are eligible to claim this benefit to supplement their income.

142

Financial, employment and legal problems

Rent and rates rebates
Old people may be entitled to a range of other allowances, including rent and rate rebates (details under housing, Chapter 8), widow's benefit or the allowances for the disabled.

Those who are injured at work

Industrial injury benefit
Industrial injury benefit may be paid when an employee cannot work because of an industrial accident at work or a prescribed industrial disease. It is paid for 26 weeks after the accident or development of the disease and is increased if there are any dependants.

Any employed person who has an accident at work should tell his employer at once and a claim should be made.

Industrial disablement benefit
Industrial disablement benefit is paid if there is disablement due to an accident at work or a disease. The extent of any disablement is assessed by a medical board as the pension payable depends on how disabled the person is. In addition, the disabled person may claim other allowances such as the constant attendance allowance, special hardship allowance and unemployability supplement.

Industrial death benefit
If a death arises from an accident at work or a prescribed disease, a dependant may claim industrial death benefit.

For those who are handicapped or disabled

Benefits for the disabled
There are a number of non-contributory benefits which are described in greater detail in Chapter 5. They are as follows:

(1) The attendance allowance, available for the severely disabled;

(2) The invalid care allowance, for those who have to care for the severely disabled;

(3) The non-contributory invalidity pension; and

(4) The mobility allowance for those unable, or virtually unable, to walk.

In addition, families with a severely handicapped child may benefit from help obtainable from the Family Fund.

Supplementary benefit

In 1979 around 5 million people were claiming supplementary benefit. This large number is partly due to the fact that many of

143

the major benefits, such as retirement pensions, are lower than the amount deemed necessary for someone to live on.

Supplementary benefit is payable to most people aged 16 or over who have left school and who are not working. Exceptions include school leavers, students and those involved in strikes. Supplementary benefit can be claimed by anyone whose income is below a certain level and it can, therefore, be used to supplement other state benefits, such as retirement pensions or private resources. Claimants under state pension age and fit for work will usually have to register for work in order to obtain this benefit.

Cohabitation rule
Claimants are most commonly single parents, sick or disabled persons, pensioners or the unemployed. Married women or those living with a man cannot receive supplementary benefit in their own right. Thus, many women claimants, including single-parent families, risk having their benefit withdrawn if they have any regular relationship with a man, even though he does not support them.

Amount payable
The amount of supplementary benefit payable is worked out by taking a claimant's 'requirements' (e.g. rent, food, etc.) and deducting from these his 'resources' or income. The 'requirements' and 'resources' of a married couple in the same household and their children are counted together and only the husband can claim. Those who have received supplementary benefit for a continuous period of 1 year or more are entitled to slightly more money.

Extra allowances payable
In addition, a patient may be eligible for extra benefit, especially the disabled or ill. Extra allowances can be given to those on special diets or who have extra laundry costs. Some claimants are eligible for allowances towards heating costs.

Exceptional needs payments
These are also lump-sum payments of benefit called exceptional needs payments and they are particularly useful for those who have been living on supplementary benefit for some time. These payments are made where a person or family need to replace or buy costly items such as new bedding, essential furniture, household or nursery equipment. These payments can also be made for expenses involved in moving house, decorating, travelling or for funeral expenses. The claimant will be expected to use his own savings over £300 for these expenses before help is given.

Automatic entitlement to other benefits
People receiving supplementary benefit and their dependants are also exempt from paying for a number of items such as NHS charges, free school meals, free milk and vitamins for expectant mothers and children under school age.

144

Urgent cases

In a local disaster, such as a flood or a fire, the local social
security office will usually be able to help in the task of
financial relief. The social security office can also help when
someone has lost their money for some reason or if someone
is stranded away from home.

Help in an emergency

Help with financial problems

Individuals or families with financial difficulties can receive
advice and assistance from a number of agencies such as the
Citizens' Advice Bureau, a welfare rights department or office
or the DHSS. Voluntary agencies such as the Child Poverty
Action Group or the Claimants Union (for those on benefits)
may also be able to help. These agencies can check whether the
patient is receiving all the benefits for which he is eligible.

Agencies who can advise and assist

For those with large debts and arrears, more intensive help
may be necessary, including help with budgeting. A social
worker from the social services department may be able to help,
or a social worker from a voluntary agency such as Family
Service Units or the Family Welfare Association. Those on
benefits who find it difficult to manage their money can arrange
for their rent to be paid directly by the DHSS or have gas or
electricity meters installed.

Budgeting help

Fuel or rent direct

Charitable organizations are often willing to help those in
financial need. Charities linked to specific disabilities or
occupations are likely to be helpful depending on the patient's
circumstances. Social workers should be knowledgeable of the
best ones to approach and are often willing to do this on the
patient's behalf.

Help from charities

Employment problems

The importance of employment

Most people need to work for a living to provide for their own
personal needs and those of their dependants. More women are
now working and make up a large section of the total work
force, contributing largely to the family income.

However, apart from the financial aspect, work provides an
occupation for much of the day and is a convenient way to
make friends and acquaintances. It is also important to an

Social aspects of work

individual's self-esteem and feelings of 'worth' and can give prestige and personal satisfaction.

Effects of job dissatisfaction

Unhappiness at work can lead to a patient showing signs of stress, depression or psychosomatic illness. This can be due to a job being boring, repetitive or due to poor working conditions. Alternatively, the job may be too demanding or stressful. Poor relationships at work may also lead to job dissatisfaction.

The psychological effects of unemployment

Unemployment can also bring distress and psychosomatic symptoms. The unemployed person may feel that there is a great stigma attached to being unemployed and having to claim benefit. There is usually a fall in living standards, the individual or family finding it difficult to cope on the reduced income.

Long-term unemployment

Long-term unemployment can be particularly demoralizing and the individual concerned may feel that he has no proper role in society. Men, in particular, may find it difficult to adjust to having no occupation and being at home all day. They may quickly become bored with nothing to do. This may lead to

Social isolation

social isolation, as the individual is often too demoralized to meet former friends and acquaintances or does not have the money to go out. Many unemployed may find it difficult to admit that they have lost their job or may have been made redundant. These problems will inevitably put stresses and strains on family life and the marital relationship.

Youth unemployment

Unemployment among the young can be particularly distressing. The school leaver usually looks forward to having a job, some money to spend and the independence which goes with it. Having nothing to do can lead to frustration and aimlessness. The young person may become depressed and isolated or give vent to his anger by turning to vandalism, hostility towards others or crime.

Services available

Department of Employment

The Department of Employment has central responsibility for most services connected with working, the local authorities playing a relatively small role.

Employment offices or job centres

Information regarding job vacancies can be obtained from employment offices or job centres. There is usually a self-service area where job details are displayed on cards and people can choose for themselves. If there are any jobs of interest, the receptionist will make an appointment with the employer.

Financial, employment and legal problems

Employment
officers can
advise

Specialist
services

In addition, there are employment advisers who will discuss job opportunities and give advice. Employment offices also offer specialist help. This includes the rehabilitation and resettlement service to cater for the disabled, advice on training, and services for particular categories of jobs such as shop and office workers, nursing, hotel and catering, etc. There are also a number of specialist branches for professional men and women and executives (Professional and Executive Recruitment) and a service for people leaving the Armed Services.

Taking a job in another area

Schemes to
increase job
mobility

There are two schemes to assist the search for jobs in other areas, thus increasing job mobility. The employment transfer scheme provides financial help to unemployed workers to take up work in places beyond travelling distance from their homes. The job search schemes also make grants to the unemployed for travel expenses to new areas to find work.

Private employment agencies

Private
agencies

Apart from statutory agencies there are a number of private agencies which often specialize in particular kinds of employment, e.g. nursing, managerial and secretarial work. Newspaper periodicals also carry advertisements for certain jobs.

Financial assistance for the unemployed

The unemployed can claim unemployment benefit if they have sufficient national insurance contributions. Those with no or insufficient contributions can claim supplementary benefit.

Training

Training

Individuals can receive training through their employers, from further education colleges or from professional and voluntary bodies. In addition, many people are trained by the Training Opportunities Schemes run by the government (TOPS).

TOPS is intended to complement training given by employers, by providing individuals with the opportunity to learn new

147

The training
opportunity
scheme

skills or update existing ones, thus enhancing their employment prospects. The scheme is open to the unemployed, to
employed people wishing to change their occupations, and to
those seeking to return to employment after a period of
absence. Disabled people are also eligible.

A weekly training allowance is paid to TOPS trainees which
is increased if there are dependants. Certain expenses are also
paid. Details of TOPS courses and the allowances available can
be obtained from employment offices or job centres.

Youth employment

The transition from school to work is an important event in a
person's life and the choice of a first job is especially important;
therefore guidance is often necessary.

Careers
teachers and
careers
officers

Most secondary schools have career teachers to advise school
leavers on employment prospects and further education.
Careers officers are also appointed by local authorities to help.
They advise young people on job vacancies and training
opportunities. Careers officers normally interview each applicant and advise them on the best course to pursue. Job centres
also employ a youth employment officer who can help.

Unemployment

The young school leaver has been one of the groups most
affected by unemployment. However, the school leaver now
has a number of options. He may return to school to obtain
more education or enrol at a Further Education College to learn

Courses
available

a craft or skill. He can undertake a training course organized by
the employment office or enrol in a Job Creation Programme.
Young people over the age of 19 are eligible to apply for a TOPS

Youth
Opportunity
Programme

course. Under 19 they are eligible to take part in the Youth
Opportunity Programme (YOP) if they have been unemployed
for 6 weeks or more. This programme offers courses to prepare
for work as well as different forms of work experience.

Alternatively, young people may benefit from other
programmes administered by the Manpower Services
Commission which give them temporary jobs on projects
which benefit the community.

Problems with conditions of employment

Protection
at work

There is a series of laws which exist to protect individuals at work. They deal with sex and racial discrimination, protection against redundancy, dismissal, industrial injuries, and health and safety at work. Advice and information can be obtained from a Citizens' Advice Bureau or legal centre or one of the specialized bodies included in the Appendices.

Legal problems

This subject is too complex to be covered at any length in this book. However, patients with legal problems can receive initial advice on whom to contact by visiting the Citizens' Advice Bureau who have lists of solicitors operating in the area. The Citizens' Advice Bureau will also know if there is a local legal advice or law centre. In these centres, lawyers offer free advice and sometimes a limited amount of further assistance.

Legal advice
and law
centres

Legal aid and legal advice and assistance

This is a scheme by which people on low incomes can receive the help of a solicitor without paying the full amount. It is administered by the Law Society and payment is related to income. Legal aid is free to people on family income supplement or on supplementary benefit.

Legal aid

Basically, there are three different schemes. First, the 'green form' scheme allows the client to get advice from a solicitor, exclusive of any court appearance. Secondly, civil legal aid covers advice and representation for a court case. Thirdly, there is criminal legal aid for defence in a criminal case.

Summary of the services and help available

Agency	*Type of help*

Financial problems

Agency	Type of help
Local office of the Department of Health and Social Security	Financial help for many sections of the population including widows, the unemployed, single parent families, pensioners, the disabled and those on low incomes (see Table 3)
	Financial help in an emergency

(post offices often have leaflets with details of benefits and application forms)

Agency	Type of help
Local authority housing department	Financial help to those on low incomes through rate or rent rebate/allowances
Department of Education	Financial help to low income families to help with the costs of schooling
Local authority social services department	Financial help to families (usually in exceptional circumstances)
	Social work assistance for those with large debts
Voluntary organizations	Financial help (a social worker may help to apply for such aid)

Advice can be obtained from Citizens' Advice Bureaux, welfare rights officers (often in the town hall), the Child Poverty Action Group and the Claimants Union. Voluntary Agencies (e.g. Family Services units or the Family Welfare Association) may help with budgeting.

150

Summary of services and help available (continued)

Employment and legal problems

Local employment offices (Department of Employment)

Advice on careers (Youth Employment Office)

Advice on job vacancies as well as details

A range of specialist services for certain job categories or for the disabled

Training courses for adults (TOPS courses)

A Youth Opportunity Programme for unemployed school leavers

Advice on careers can also be obtained from the careers teachers at school or the careers officers appointed by the local authority (education department).

Legal aid and advice can be obtained from law centres, legal advice centres as well as from solicitors. The Citizens' Advice Bureau is usually a good starting point as it will give initial advice as well as having details of schemes and solicitors in the area.

Appendix 1 General co-ordinating bodies and sources of information

NATIONAL ASSOCIATION OF CITIZENS' ADVICE BUREAUX
110 Drury Lane, London WC2B 5SW (01 836 9231). There are more than 500 local offices, the addresses of which can be found in the telephone directory, town hall, library or post office.

CHARITY COMMISSION
St Alban's House, 57–60 Haymarket, London SW1Y 4QX (01 214 6000). Alphabetical, geographical and functional national index of charities. Open to public inspection.

NATIONAL COUNCIL OF SOCIAL SERVICE
26 Bedford Square, London WC1B 3HU (01 636 4066). This is the national co-ordinating body of the local councils of social service and it will have details of the addresses of local councils of social service.

For Scotland, Wales and Northern Ireland:
Scottish Council for Social Service, 18/19 Claremont Crescent, Edinburgh EH7 4HX (031 556 3882).
Council of Social Service for Wales, 2 Cathedral Road, Cardiff CF1 9XR (0222 21456).
Northern Ireland Council for Social Service, 2 Annandale Avenue, Belfast BT7 3JH (0232 643886).

Appendix 2 Voluntary organizations: children and young people

CHURCH OF ENGLAND CHILDREN'S SOCIETY

Old Town Hall, Kennington Road, London SE11 4QD (01 735 2441). Provides advice and casework support to families in need and operates an adoption and fostering service. It runs 67 child care centres, including residential schools and homes for the handicapped.

DR BARNADO'S

Tanner's Lane, Barkingside, Ilford, Essex 1G6 1QG (01 550 8822). Provides care and treatment for children in need, both residential and non-residential, including facilities for the physically and mentally handicapped.

FAMILY SERVICE UNITS

207 Old Marylebone Road, London NW1 5QP (01 402 5175). There are local branches throughout the country. The units give practical assistance and counselling to families unable to cope.

FAMILY WELFARE ASSOCIATION

501–3 Kingsland Road, London E8 4AU (01 254 6251). There are over 100 of these organizations which give counselling and practical help to families. Only a few of them are called Family Welfare Associations but the Citizens' Advice Bureau or the central office of the FWA will have the address of the nearest agency.

NATIONAL CHILDREN'S HOME

85 Highbury Park, London N5 1UD (01 226 2033). Has a number of residential homes for children as well as schools or day care facilities. It also caters for the physically and mentally handicapped. It provides financial and housing aid, is involved in adoption work and runs playgroups.

NATIONAL SOCIETY FOR THE PREVENTION OF CRUELTY TO CHILDREN (NSPCC)

1 Riding House Street, London W1P 8AA (01 580 8812). There are 200 or more branches of this society. They carry out a range of preventive work with families as well as assessing and helping potential or actual 'child abuse' cases.

PARENTS ANONYMOUS

9 Manor Gardens, Islington, London N7 (01 263 8918). A 24 hour telephone service offering help to parents in the Greater London area who may feel tempted to abuse their children. Helpers are volunteers who have had in-service training.

NATIONAL YOUTH BUREAU

17/23 Albion Street, Leicester LE1 6GD (0533 538811). This gives detailed information about local recreational schemes and youth clubs. The National Association of Young People's Counselling and Advisory schemes, which has details of local counselling agencies for the young, are also at the same address and phone number.

YOUNG MEN'S CHRISTIAN ASSOCIATION

640 Forest Road, London E17 3DZ (01 520 5599).

YOUNG WOMEN'S CHRISTIAN ASSOCIATION

2 Weymouth Street, London W1N 4AX (01 636 9722). These organizations run youth clubs and provide hostel accommodation in most large towns and cities.

TASK FORCE

1 Thorpe Close, off Cambridge Gardens, London W10 5XL (01 960 5669). Organizes young volunteers to visit and give practical help to lonely and housebound elderly people.

Appendix 3 Voluntary organizations: adult and family life

NATIONAL MARRIAGE GUIDANCE COUNCIL
Little Church Street, Rugby, Warwickshire. (0788 73241). There are 150 local marriage guidance councils giving help to those with marital difficulties.

JEWISH MARRIAGE EDUCATION COUNCIL
529B Finchley Road, London NW3 7BG (01 794 8035). Gives advice and help to Jews with marital difficulties.

CATHOLIC MARRIAGE GUIDANCE COUNCIL
Clitherow House, 15 Landsdowne Road, London W11 3AJ (01 727 0141). There are 60 centres to help Catholics with marital or psychosexual problems.

FAMILY PLANNING ASSOCIATION
27–35 Mortimer Street, London W1N 7RJ (01 636 7866). Some of the branches offer psychosexual counselling as well as contraceptive advice and sex education.

NATIONAL WOMEN'S AID FEDERATION
374 Grays Inn Road, London WC1 (01 837 9316). This has over 100 affiliated groups offering help and temporary accommodation for women and their children who have been suffering mental or physical violence.
Welsh Women's Aid, Adams Street, Cardiff (0222 388291).
Scottish Women's Aid, 11 St Colme Street, Edinburgh EH3 6AA (031 225 8011).

NATIONAL COUNCIL FOR ONE PARENT FAMILIES

255 Kentish Town Road, London NW5 2LX (01 267 1361). Gives sympathetic advice and practical help to single parents, including representation at tribunals, and publishes informative pamphlets and booklets.

(Also the Scottish Council for Single Parents, 44 Albany Street, Edinburgh EH1 3QR (031 556 3899).

GINGERBREAD

35 Wellington House, London WC2 (01 240 0953). There are 300 local groups operating on the self-help principle, giving advice, practical help and providing social activities for single-parent families.

BROOK ADVISORY CENTRES

153a East Street, London SE17 2SD (01 708 1234). This centre and others provide counselling on emotional and sexual problems for young people as well as advice on birth control or termination of pregnancy.

BRITISH PREGNANCY ADVISORY SERVICE

Austy Manor, Wootten Warren, Solihull, W. Midlands. B95 6DA (Henley in Arden) (05642 3225).

PREGNANCY ADVISORY SERVICES

40 Margaret Street, London W1N 7FB (01 409 0281). These organizations give advice and can make arrangements for termination of pregnancy at moderate fees. The British Pregnancy Advisory Service has a number of branches offering a counselling service over the telephone.

NATIONAL ASSOCIATION FOR THE WIDOWED AND THEIR CHILDREN (CRUSE)

126 Sheen Road, Richmond, Surrey TW9 1UR (01 940 4818). Local Cruse clubs aim to help widows and widowers through advisory services, counselling, parents' circles, etc.

INTERNATIONAL SOCIAL SERVICE OF GREAT BRITAIN

Cranmer House, 39 Brixton Road, London SW9 6DD (01 735 8941). Helps with personal and family problems extending across national frontiers.

GAY SWITCHBOARD

(01 837 7324). A telephone information and advice service for homosexual men and women run by carefully selected volunteers. There are a number of other organizations nation-wide.

APEX TRUST

31–3 Clapham Road, London SW9 0JE (01 582 3171). Offers employment and information services for ex-offenders.

NATIONAL ASSOCIATION FOR THE CARE AND RESETTLEMENT OF OFFENDERS (NACRO)

169 Clapham Road, London SW9 0PU (01 582 6500). Provides an advice and information service and co-ordinates a number of local associations working for prisoners and their families.

NATIONAL COUNCIL FOR THE SINGLE WOMAN AND HER DEPENDANTS

29 Chilworth Mews, London W2 3RG (01 262 1451). Assists single women with elderly or infirm dependants. It has 40 branches.

ASSOCIATION OF BRITISH ADOPTION AND FOSTERING AGENCIES

11 Southwark Street, London SE1 1RQ (01 407 8800). Has details of adoption and fostering agencies.

NATIONAL FEDERATION OF SOLO CLUBS

7–8 Ruskin Chambers, 191 Corporation Street, Birmingham B4 (021 236 2879). Provides details of clubs for single, separated or divorced people.

Appendix 4 Voluntary organizations: the elderly

AGE CONCERN ENGLAND

(National Old People's Welfare Council) Bernard Sunley House, 60 Pitcairn Road, Mitcham, Surrey CR4 3LL (01 640 5431). Age Concern is the focal point for more than 1500 old people's welfare organizations. The national body provides an information and advice service on all aspects of the welfare of the elderly.

LOCAL AGE CONCERN (OLD PEOPLE'S WELFARE) ORGANIZATIONS

Some of the activities and services which may be provided through the local groups of Age Concern (Old People's Welfare) are: good neighbour and street warden schemes; personal help with shopping; hairdressing or decorating; advice on welfare rights; grants for heating and heating appliances; transport by car or special bus; holidays; outings and entertainment and many others. The address of a local organization is available from the appropriate social services department, Citizens' Advice Bureau, and other advice and information centres.

COUNSEL AND CARE FOR THE ELDERLY (ELDERLY INVALIDS FUND)

131 Middlesex Street, London E1 7JF (01 621 1624). Provides an information and advisory service on all matters of concern to elderly people. The CCE arrange financial help in cases of need.

THE EMPLOYMENT FELLOWSHIP

Drayton House, Gordon Street, London WC1H OBE (01 387 1828). The Fellowship is a small charity whose principal object is to encourage and assist in the setting up of sheltered work centres for the elderly. At present there are over 150 such centres in the UK providing employment for over 6000 old age pensioners.

HELP THE AGED

32 Dover Street, London W1A 2AP (01 449 0972). This is an international organization for the relief of distress amongst old people, both in the United Kingdom and overseas. It actively promotes day centres, workshops, housing and day hospitals for the elderly

DISTRESSED GENTLEFOLK'S AID ASSOCIATION

Vicarage Gate House, Vicarage Gate, London W8 (01 229 9341). Provides financial help, clothing, comforts and holidays in suitable cases. It also runs a number of residential homes with nursing care.

WOMEN'S ROYAL VOLUNTARY SERVICE

17 Old Park Lane, London W1Y 4AJ (01 499 6040). Carries out a wide range of work for all sections of the community, including the elderly and handicapped. Local groups may provide visiting schemes, playgroups, second-hand clothing, social clubs for the elderly, holiday schemes, distribution of welfare foods, meals-on-wheels, housing schemes and transport.

THE PRE-RETIREMENT ASSOCIATION

19 Undine Street, London SW17 8PP (01 767 3225). The Association is primarily concerned to focus attention on the need to prepare for retirement and to remain active and involved when employment has ceased. It will have details on courses available.

Appendix 5 Voluntary organizations: the physically disabled

This appendix includes only a small proportion of the agencies available to help the handicapped.

THE DISABLED LIVING FOUNDATION

346 Kensington High Street, London W14 8NS (01 602 2491). Provides a comprehensive information service for the disabled run on a subscription basis. The Foundation also has an aids centre with a permanent exhibition.

DISABLED INCOME GROUP (DIG)

Attlee House, 28 Commercial Street, London E1 6LR (01 247 218). DIG is a pressure group with local branches campaigning for legislative reform to provide adequate income and allowances for disabled.

DISABILITY ALLIANCE

1 Cambrige Terrace, London NW1 4JL (01 935 4992). The Alliance is a federation of organizations for the disabled which aims to achieve a comprehensive income scheme for disabled people.

THE ROYAL ASSOCIATION FOR DISABILITY AND REHABILITATION (RADAR)

25 Mortimer Street, London W1N 8AB (01 637 5400). RADAR is a co-ordinating body with more than 300 affiliated voluntary organizations. It acts as an information bureau and is concerned with every aspect of physical disability.

BRITISH RED CROSS

9 Grosvenor Crescent, London SW1X 7EJ (01 235 7131). Offers a wide variety of services in hospitals and in people's homes. These include nursing services, loans of aids and gadgets, home visiting, social clubs, residential homes, holidays, providing escorts and first aid.

BRITISH SPORTS ASSOCIATION FOR THE DISABLED

Hayward House, Harvey Road, Aylesbury, Bucks. HP21 8PP (0296 27889) organizes sports meetings, lectures and demonstrations for the disabled. It has a number of regional committees.

Organizations for more specific illnesses

ARTHRITIS CARE (THE BRITISH RHEUMATISM AND ARTHRITIS ASSOCIATION)

6 Grosvenor Crescent, London SW1X 7ER (01 235 0902). The Association has over 200 branches which provide basic information about welfare services, allowances, aids for the disabled and holidays.

ASSOCIATION FOR SPINA BIFIDA AND HYDRO-CEPHALUS (ASBAH)

Tavistock House North, Tavistock Square, London SW1H 9HJ (01 388 1382/5). Gives support, advice, including help with holidays, equipment, training, employment and welfare grants. There are some 80 local associations in England, Wales and Northern Ireland, also Scottish Spina Bifida Association, 190 Queensbury Road, Edinburgh EH4 2BW (031 322 0743).

ASSOCIATION TO COMBAT HUNTINGTON'S CHOREA

Lyndhurst, Lower Hampton Road, Sunbury-on-Thames, Middlesex, TW16 5PR (01 979 5055). Provides help of all kinds to those affected with this hereditary disease. It has 18 branches throughout Britain.

BRITISH DIABETIC ASSOCIATION

10 Queen Anne Street, London W1M 0AE (01 558 4064). Provides diabetics with information, advice and holidays for diabetic children. It publishes a bi-monthly newspaper, cassette recordings of which are available to the registered blind.

THE BRITISH EPILEPSY ASSOCIATION
Crowthorne House, New Wokingham Road, Wokingham, Berkshire RG11 3AY (Crowthorne) (0344 3122); Regional Office: 44 Eastgate, Leeds LS2 7SL (0532 454416). This provides an advisory and an holiday service. There are some 80 Action for Epilepsy groups in the country.

CHEST, HEART AND STROKE ASSOCIATION
Tavistock House North, Tavistock Square, London WC1H 9JE (01 387 3012). Carries our research, health education, rehabilitation, welfare and counselling services.

THE MULTIPLE SCLEROSIS SOCIETY OF GREAT BRITAIN AND NORTHERN IRELAND
286 Munster Road, London SW6 6BE (01 381 4022). The Society has some 270 local branches providing a free counselling service, outings, holidays, social activities and financial help to sufferers and their families.

MUSCULAR DYSTROPHY GROUP OF GREAT BRITAIN
Nattrass House, 35 Macaulay Road, London SW4 0QP (01 720 8055). As well as a number of research centres, the Group also provides services and social contacts through over 300 local branches.

NATIONAL SOCIETY FOR CANCER RELIEF
30 Dorset Square, London NW1 6QL (01 402 8125). The Society provides financial assistance to help any heavy debts, nursing and convalescent home fees, day or night nursing, fares for relatives visiting patients in hospital etc., and a basic weekly grant for everyday necessities to patients in conjunction with the NHS. The Society is building a network of 'continuing care units' to provide specialist care for in-patients and out-patients (also the Marie Curie Memorial Foundation).

PARKINSON'S DISEASE SOCIETY
81 Queens Road, London SW19 8NR (01 946 2500). Aims to help patients and their relatives with problems in the home, to collect and disseminate information, and to sponsor research into the disease.

ROYAL BRITISH LEGION

48–9 Pall Mall, London SW1Y 5JY (01 930 8131). The Legion is particularly concerned with the welfare of ex-service personnel and their dependants, e.g. in areas of employment and rehabilitation, housing, financial benefits, grants, allowances and pensions. It runs several country homes for aged or infirm ex-servicemen, convalescent homes and a number of factories providing sheltered employment.

THE SPASTICS SOCIETY

12 Park Crescent, London W1N 4EQ (01 636 5020). Aims to provide care, treatment, education and employment training for spastics. The Society has established more than 160 schools and centres and provides a comprehensive range of services and opportunities. Also the Scottish Council for Spastics, 22 Corstorphine Road, Edinburgh EH12 6HP (031 337 9876).

The blind and partially sighted

THE PARTIALLY SIGHTED SOCIETY

40 Wandsworth Road, Hove, East Sussex BN3 5BH (0273 736053) provides information on aids, careers and employment available to partially sighted people.

THE ROYAL NATIONAL INSTITUTE FOR THE BLIND (RNIB)

224 Great Portland Street, London W1N 6AA (01 388 1266). Promotes and facilitates education, training, rehabilitation, employment and welfare of blind people, and provides special schools, homes, training establishments, a wide range of industrial and recreational appliances and braille publications.

ST DUNSTAN'S FOR MEN AND WOMEN BLINDED ON WAR SERVICE

191 Old Marylebone Road, London NW1 5QN (01 723 5021). Provides training, resettlement and aftercare for men and women blinded on active service with the armed forces or with civil defence services, e.g. police and fire services.

GUIDE DOGS FOR THE BLIND ASSOCIATION

9–11 Park Street, Windsor, Berkshire (07535 55711). Provides guide dogs and training facilities for blind people aged between 18 and 60 years.

The deaf and hard of hearing

THE BREAKTHROUGH TRUST

Charles W. Gillett Centre, Selly Oak Colleges, Birmingham
B29 6LE (021 472 6447). The aim of the Trust is to integrate
deaf with hearing people by means of self-help groups.

THE ROYAL NATIONAL INSTITUTE FOR THE DEAF (RNID)

105 Gower Street, London WC1E 6AH (01 387 8033). Runs
several residential establishments including a training centre
and a special school. It also provides a comprehensive information and advisory service with a library and technical department. (Scottish Association for the Deaf, Moray House,
Edinburgh EH8 8AQ (031 556 8137)).

THE BRITISH DEAF ASSOCIATION

38 Victoria Place, Carlisle CA1 1HU (0228 20188). Has many
branches. It organizes a variety of group activities for deaf
people and is able to advise individuals and parents on
development and education. It provides residential care and
financial assistance.

THE BRITISH ASSOCIATION OF THE HARD OF HEARING

6 Great James Street, London WC1N 3DA (01 405 5182). There
are over 200 local groups in the United Kingdom providing a
wide range of educational, cultural and social activities.

NATIONAL DEAF CHILDREN'S SOCIETY

45 Hereford Road, London W2 5AH (01 229 9272/6). Aims to
improve and advance the arrangements for the education of
deaf and partially hearing children. It operates through local
groups of parents of deaf children.

The deaf–blind

THE NATIONAL DEAF–BLIND HELPERS' LEAGUE

18 Rainbow Court, Paston Ridings, Peterborough, PE4 6UP
(0733 73511). Provides social activities in local groups. It also
provides private self-contained flats for the independent deaf–
blind and some holiday accommodation.

THE NATIONAL ASSOCIATION FOR DEAF–BLIND AND RUBELLA HANDICAPPED

164 Cromwell Lane, Coventry, CV4 8AP (0203 462579). Gives advice about financial and educational problems, and support to parents.

Handicapped children

INVALID CHILDREN'S AID ASSOCIATION (ICAA)

126 Buckingham Palace Road, London SW1W 9SB (01 730 9891). The Association has an information service providing free advice for parents. It runs a number of residential schools, a social work and group work service, playgroups and a toy library.

VOLUNTARY COUNCIL FOR HANDICAPPED CHILDREN

8 Wakley Street, Islington, London EC1V 7QE (01 278 9441). Provides an information service to parents and professionals and has details on the voluntary agencies which can help.

ASSOCIATION OF PARENTS OF VACCINE DAMAGED CHILDREN

2 Church Street, Shipston-on-Stour, Warwickshire CU36 4AP (0608 61595). This organization represents, through parents, the children who have suffered handicaps as a result of vaccination.

ASSOCIATION OF ALL SPEECH IMPAIRED CHILDREN

347 Central Market, Smithfield, London EC1A 9NH (01 236 3632). Provides advisory and information services for children with speech impairments.

BREAK (DAVISON MORLEY TRUST)

20 Hooks Hill Road, Sheringham, Norfolk NR26 8NL (0263 823170). Provides holidays, short-term, long-term, and emergency care for the handicapped and the deprived child.

Appendix 6 Voluntary organizations: the mentally disordered

MIND (THE NATIONAL ASSOCIATION FOR MENTAL HEALTH)

22 Harley Street, London W1N 2ED (01 637 0741). MIND seeks to improve services for the mentally disordered. It runs an advisory service offering advice, referral and short-term help to patients and their families. It has a legal and welfare rights service to protect the rights of patients and mental health social workers and to press for changes in the law. MIND has also pioneered a number of residential schools, homes and hostels for children and adults.

MENCAP (THE NATIONAL SOCIETY FOR MENTALLY HANDICAPPED CHILDREN AND ADULTS)

117 Golden Lane, London EC1Y 0RT (01 253 9433). This Society has over 450 local branches and 12 regional offices providing help and advice for mentally handicapped people. The Society aims to improve the provision for mentally handicapped children and adults especially by increasing public knowledge and concern. It runs special holidays for children and adults and has residential homes. It also helps to organize local services, special care units, clubs, creches and emergency care facilities. Recent developments include speech therapy and physiotherapy advisory services. MENCAP runs social activities and employment training courses for young mentally handicapped adults and operates a trustee insurance scheme.

RICHMOND FELLOWSHIP

8 Addison Road, London W14 8DL (01 603 6373). The Fellowship provides residential short-term and long-term therapeutic care for people who have suffered and are on the verge of a nervous breakdown.

BRITISH ASSOCIATION OF COUNSELLING

1a Cuttle Church Street, Rugby, Warwickshire CO21 3AP (0788 78328). It has published a directory of agencies offering therapy, counselling and support in psychosexual problems.

MENTAL AFTER-CARE ASSOCIATION

Eagle House, 110 Jermyn Street, London SW1Y 6HB (01 839 5953). The Association provides hostels for the rehabilitation of people after discharge from mental hospital, and homes for those requiring long-term care.

PARENTS FOR CHILDREN

222 Camden High Street, London NW1 8QR (01 485 7526). This voluntary organization operates in London and the Home Counties. It specializes in finding homes for hard to place children.

NATIONAL SCHIZOPHRENIA FELLOWSHIP

78 Victoria Street, Surbiton, Surrey (01 390 3651). This 'self-help' organization gives advice, support and help to schizophrenic patients and their relatives. There are over 150 local groups.

SAMARITANS

17 Uxbridge Road, Slough, Berkshire SL1 1SN (0753 32713). This organization has a branch office in most localities and normally runs a 24 hour telephone answering service, volunteers giving sympathy and advice to anyone who rings. The centres are often open to people who wish to call in person during office hours. Some areas also run special services for those with sexual problems.

EX-SERVICES MENTAL WELFARE SOCIETY

37–9 Thurloe Street, London SW7 2LL (01 584 8688). This society assists ex-members of the forces suffering from mental disorders.

ALCOHOLICS ANONYMOUS

11 Redcliffe Gardens, London SW10 9BG (01 352 9669). A self-help organization for alcoholics. Alcoholics are befriended and can call their befriender when needing help. They are also helped by attending one or more groups offering group therapy.

AL-ANON FAMILY GROUPS

61 Great Dover Street, London SE1 4YF (01 403 0888). Offers group support and friendship for relatives of problem drinkers. There are local groups throughout the country and a number of them give support specifically to teenagers (aged 12–20) with an alcoholic friend or relative (Alateen).

GAMBLERS ANONYMOUS AND GAM-ANON

17–23 Blantyre St. Cheyne Walk, London SW10 (01 352 3060). As with alcoholics anonymous, group therapy is an important part of this agency's help for those with gambling problems. Practical help and advice is given.

HELPING HAND ORGANIZATION

8 Strutton Ground, London SW1P 2HP (01 222 8862). Provides residential homes for the rehabilitation of those suffering from drug or alcohol dependence and for young people at risk. It also offers a counselling service.

THE PHOBICS SOCIETY

4 Cheltenham Road, Chorlton-cum-Hardy, Manchester M21 1QN (061 881 1937). This is a self-help pressure group. Groups exist throughout the country to help sufferers.

RELEASE

1 Elgin Avenue, London W9 3PR (01 289 1123). Provides legal, medical and social information about drug addiction.

Appendix 7 Voluntary organizations: housing problems

THE INSTITUTE OF HOUSING
Victoria House, Southampton Row, London WC1B 4EB (01 242 3267). Has a list of housing aid or advice centres.

THE HOUSING CORPORATION
149 Tottenham Court Road, London W1P 0BN (01 387 9466).

NATIONAL FEDERATION OF HOUSING ASSOCIATIONS
30–32 Southampton Street, Strand, London WC2E 7HE (01 240 2771). These organizations can give advice and assistance about housing associations.

THE CAMPAIGN FOR HOMELESS AND ROOTLESS (CHAR)
27 John Adam Street, London WC2 (01 839 6185). Co-ordinates the work of many of the organizations for the single homeless and can give advice.

THE ADVISORY SERVICE FOR SQUATTERS
2 St Paul's Road, London N1 (01 359 8814). Gives advice on squatting and homelessness.

SHELTER
157 Walterloo Road, London SE1 8UU (01 633 9377). Gives advice and help to families with any kind of housing problem.

NATIONAL CYRENIANS
13 Wincheap, Canterbury, Kent CT1 3TB (0227 51641). Provides residential homes, night shelters and day centres for the single homeless.

Appendix 8 Voluntary organizations: financial, employment and legal problems

CHILD POVERTY ACTION GROUP
1 Macklin Street, London WC2 (01 242 3225). Provides relief of poverty among children and families and advises on welfare rights problems. The group publishes the National Welfare Benefits Handbook, a very useful guide.

NATIONAL FEDERATION OF CLAIMANTS' UNION
Local groups support and advise those on supplementary benefit.

REGULAR FORCES EMPLOYMENT ASSOCIATION
25 Bloomsbury Square, London WC1A 2LN (01 637 3918). The Association has a number of branches and aims to provide suitable employment for men and women leaving the services.

SOLDIERS', SAILORS' AND AIRMEN'S FAMILIES ASSOCIATION
27 Queen Anne's Gate, London SW1H 9BZ (01 222 9221). Provides a general welfare and advisory service to families of serving, ex-servicemen and women and has over 1000 branches.

NATIONAL COUNCIL FOR CIVIL LIBERTIES
186 Kings Cross Road, London WC1X 9DE (01 278 4575). Gives legal advice to protect the rights and liberties of the private citizen, especially minority groups.

Index